Understanding the Impact of Clergy Sexual Abuse

The sexual exploitation of a child by one who has been recognized as a representative of God is a sinister assault on that person's psychosocial and spiritual well-being. Many survivors of such abuse present with a range of symptoms consistent with Posttraumatic Stress Disorder as well as common co-occurring problems, including substance abuse, affective lability, and relational conflicts. Yet there are additional themes, particularly the impact of the abuse and institutional betrayal on the family, profound alteration in individual spirituality, and changes in individual and family religious practices, which differentiate this abuse from other traumas.

Understanding the profound and multidimensional effects of clergy perpetrated sexual abuse and the betrayal of trust by religious leaders on individuals, families and communities requires the collective wisdom of many voices. This book brings together the perspectives of survivors, practitioners and scholars to examine this unique form of interpersonal violence from theoretical, clinical and spiritual perspectives with consideration given to future research needs.

This book was published as a special issue of the *Journal of Child Sex Abuse*.

Robert A. McMackin works with the Massachusetts Department of Public Health at Lemuel Shattuck Hospital in Boston and is a member of the Tufts University School of Medicine clinical faculty.

Terence M. Keane is Director of the National Center for PTSD-Behavioral Sciences Division and Associate Chief of Staff for Research & Development at VA Boston Healthcare System. He is Professor and Vice Chairman in the Division of Psychiatry at Boston University School of Medicine. He is also Professor of Clinical Psychology at BU.

Paul M. Kline has worked in the field of child and family mental health for many years. He is an Associate Professor in the Graduate School of Social Work at Boston College where he teaches courses concerned with the care of children and families coping with violence and mental illness.

Understanding the Impact of Clergy Sexual Abuse

Betrayal and Recovery

Edited by Robert A. McMackin, Terence M. Keane and Paul M. Kline

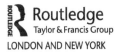
Routledge
Taylor & Francis Group

LONDON AND NEW YORK

First published 2009 by Routledge
2 Park Square, Milton Park, Abingdon, Oxon, OX14 4RN

Simultaneously published in the USA and Canada by Routledge
52 Vanderbilt Avenue, New York, NY 10017

Routledge is an imprint of the Taylor & Francis Group, an informa business

© 2009 Edited by Robert A. McMackin, Terence M. Keane and Paul M. Kline

Typeset in Times by Value Chain, India

British Library Cataloguing in Publication Data
A catalogue record for this book is available from the British Librar

ISBN13: 978-0-7890-3599-8 (hbk)
ISBN13: 978-0-7890-3600-1 (pbk)

CONTENTS

Acknowledgments

The guest editors thank the survivors, the parents and loved ones of survivors, and the clergy and mental health professionals who have been so generous in sharing their stories and wisdom. We thank William Barry, SJ, PhD, editor of *Human Development* magazine, for his early support of this project and his steady encouragement. Finally, the guest editors thank Barbara Thorp, MSW, Director of the Archdiocese of Boston Office of Pastoral Support and Outreach, for her unwavering commitment to justice and healing for survivors and their families.

About the Contributors

Stephen Brady, PhD, is Associate Professor of Psychiatry and the Director of the Mental Health and Behavioral Medicine Program at the Boston University School of Medicine. He has longstanding clinical and research interests in gay identity development, and HIV prevention and psychiatric disorders.

Stephanie Clarke received her B.A. in psychology from Smith College in 2002 and was a research technician at the Women's Health Sciences Division of the National Center for Posttraumatic Stress Disorder at the time this manuscript was submitted for publication. She is currently a graduate student in the Developmental Psychopathology and Clinical Science doctoral program at the University of Minnesota, Twin Cities. Her interests include the psychological sequelae of early social deprivation and child maltreatment with an emphasis on emotion regulation, attachment, and borderline personality symptomatology.

Kathryn A. Flynn, PhD, is currently an Associate Professor in Program Evaluation at the Defense Language Institute, Presidio of Monterey. She holds a Bachelor's Degree in Political Science from Duquesne University; a Master's Degree in Public Administration from San Diego State University; a Master's Degree in Education, and a PhD in Education from Claremont Graduate University, where she is also a Research Associate. Her research interests include a variety of topics including clergy sex abuse as it relates to women's lives; the American educational presence in early twentieth century China; and Program Evaluation related to foreign language learning.

Jason M. Fogler earned his PhD in 2005 from Boston University's Clinical Psychology Program and was a NIMH-sponsored postdoctoral fellow in a joint appointment at Boston Medical Center and the National Center for Posttraumatic Stress Disorder at the time this manuscript was submitted for publication. Dr. Fogler has studied the effects of Trauma Systems Therapy, a novel treatment for traumatized children, and the factor structure of Axis I and II disorders in a veterans' population. He is currently a clinical associate at the Brookline Community Mental Health Center in Brookline, MA, where he specializes in the treatment of traumatized children and adults.

James Freiburger, PhD, is a psychologist and owner/director of private practices in Wisconsin. In addition to specializing with survivors and perpetrators of sexual abuse, he provides forensic evaluation, testing, and testimony, workshops and seminars, and consultation and supervision to multiple agencies and corporations.

Linda Harvey has been a social worker for 45 years, has started over 50 organizations to meet human needs, and has been a mediator for 16 years in traditional, transformative, and restorative justice with civil, criminal, and church cases such as homicide, family, juveniles, child protection, clergy abuse, and human rights. In addition, she is a facilitator, trainer, and journalist. She is presently serving on the Advisory Council of the University of Kentucky College of Social Work and is Chair of the Advisory Council for the Center for the Study of Violence Against Children in Lexington, KY.

Paul J. Isely, EdD, has a doctorate in Counseling Psychology from Boston University and is currently a management consultant specializing in organizational change and strategy. Prior to this work, he was a therapist and crisis clinician, specializing in the treatment of sexual abuse. He has published several research and treatment articles on male sexual assault survivors.

Peter Isely, MA, is the Midwest Director of The Survivors Network of those Abused by Priests (SNAP) and a survivor of childhood sexual abuse by a Wisconsin priest. A graduate of Harvard Divinity School and a clinical social worker, Peter founded and operated the only inpatient program for victims of clergy sexual trauma in the country at Rogers Memorial Hospital outside of Madison, Wisconsin.

Fr. Joseph J. Guido, OP, STL, EdD, is a Roman Catholic priest and member of the Dominican Order. He is a psychologist with the Personal Counseling Center at Providence College, where he is also Assistant Professor of Psychology and Vice President for Mission and Ministry. In addition, he serves as a member of the Advisory Board for the Protection of Children and Young People for the Diocese of Providence, Rhode Island.

Jennifer M. Jensen received her M.A. in Psychology from Boston University in 2001. At the time this manuscript was submitted for publication, she coordinated a randomized clinical trial comparing manualized treatments for traumatized women veterans diagnosed with posttraumatic stress disorder at the Women's Health Sciences Division of the National Center for

Posttraumatic Stress Disorder. She is interested in examining variation in emotional response as a function of different psychopathological conditions and exposure to trauma.

Michael Lesher, Esq (JD, Brooklyn Law School, 1988; MA, University of Virginia, 1982), is a legal advocate for parents of abused children, incest survivors, and adult victims of Jewish clergy abuse. Mr. Lesher is a published author, essayist, columnist, and investigative journalist and public speaker. His topics include child abuse and family court, legal remedies for adult survivors of clergy, and intra familial abuse.

Daniel J. Levins, BA, holds an undergraduate degree in Forensic Psychology and is a former police officer. He is currently completing graduate study in Psychology and is a Ballet Master/Instructor at Elliot Feld Ballet Dance Company in New York City.

Edna Lezotte, D.Min, LICSW is a social worker in the Office of Pastoral Support and Outreach for the Roman Catholic Archdiocese of Boston. She is an adjunct faculty member in social work at Boston University and Salem State College and in the international program at Framingham State College.

Annette Mahoney, PhD, is a Professor of Psychology at Bowling Green State University. Her research focuses on the psychology of religion, particularly as applied to family life. Other research interests are links between marriage, parenting, and child behavior problems.

Nichole A. Murray-Swank, PhD, is an assistant professor in the School of Education and Counseling at Regis University. Her primary research and clinical interests focus on spirituality, sexual abuse, and trauma, as well as the integration of spirituality in the counseling process.

Amy Neustein, PhD (Sociology from Boston University 1981), is the daughter of a prominent Orthodox rabbi and founded the Help Us Regain the Children Legal Research and Advocacy Center in 1986. The Center collected a large database of clergy abuse cases nationwide, which was frequented by legislative aides and investigative reporters. Dr. Neustein is a published author, researcher, editor, and public spokesperson on clergy abuse in the Jewish religion.

Douglas E. Noll, Esq., is a full time peacemaker and mediator, specializing in difficult, complex, and intractable conflicts. He is an adjunct professor of law and has a Master's Degree in Peacemaking and Conflict Studies. He is the author of the books *Sex, Politics & Religion at the Office: The New Competitive Advantage* (Auberry Press, 2006) with John Boogaert; *Peacemaking: Practicing at the Intersection of Law and Human Conflict* (Cascadia, 2002); and numerous articles on peacemaking, restorative justice, conflict resolution, and mediation. He is also a mediator trainer, lecturer, and continuing education panelist. Mr. Noll was voted as one of the Best Lawyers in America in 2005 by bestlawyers.com.

Kenneth I. Pargament, PhD, is a Professor of Psychology at Bowling Green State University. His research focuses on the roles of religion and spirituality in coping with major life stressors and on the design and evaluation of spiritually integrated treatments.

Erin L. Rowe earned her B.A. from Hartwick College in 2001 and was a research technician at the Women's Health Sciences Division of the National Center for Posttraumatic Stress Disorder at the time this manuscript was submitted for publication. She is currently a project manager at the Institute on Urban Health Research at Northeastern University, where she manages a large four year grant examining a brief treatment intervention for college students and a two year pilot study of an intervention to improve medication adherence in HIV-positive patients. Her primary interests are substance abuse and trauma in minority populations.

Jillian C. Shipherd earned her PhD from the State University of New York at Buffalo in 2001 and is currently on the staff at the Women's Health Sciences Division of the National Center for Posttraumatic Stress Disorder as a Staff Psychologist. She also holds the position of Assistant Professor in the Department of Psychiatry at Boston University School of Medicine. Dr. Shipherd is devoted to understanding gender differences in trauma recovery including both mental and physical effects. Her work has a special emphasis on women's health issues and care for the transgender population.

James M. Sullivan, MSW, LICSW, is a professional social worker in Boston, MA, specializing in geriatric care at Care Advocacy and Resources for Elders (CARE).

Leslie H. Wind, PhD, is Assistant Professor at Boston College Graduate School of Social Work. She has been a professional social worker for 20 years and has devoted most of her direct practice to trauma survivors and their families. Her research centers on child and family coping and resilience in the aftermath of trauma exposure.

Introduction: Understanding the Trauma of Clergy Sexual Abuse

Robert A. McMackin
Terence M. Keane
Paul M. Kline

The sexual exploitation of a child by one who has been privileged, even anointed, as a representative of God is a sinister assault on that person's psychosocial and spiritual well-being. The impact of such a violent betrayal is amplified when the perpetrator is sheltered and supported by a larger religious community. In 2002, the Roman Catholic Church in

America was rocked by a flood of allegations of sexual abuse of children by priests. Records reveal that between 1950 and 2002, more than 10,000 individuals had come forward to report such abuse (The John Jay College Research Team, 2004). As overwhelming as that number is, survivors' personal stories of sexual assault occurring within a sacred milieu and the subsequent impact of that abuse on their later development have an even more powerful impact. These stories strongly suggest that church leaders invested far greater resources and concern in protecting the institution of the Catholic Church from scandal than in providing meaningful support and care for victims and their families. When these crimes and the abandonment of responsible care of survivors were finally brought to light, they erupted with enough force to shake the basic trust that once held local Catholic communities together. Furthermore, the confidence of Catholics in church leadership was deeply shaken.

The Archdiocese of Boston has been considered by many as the epicenter of what has become an international crisis within the Catholic Church. Over the past five years, the three editors of this volume have served as consultants to the Archdiocese on responding to the needs of survivors, their families, and parish communities. An initial review of the literature at the time the scandal broke revealed limited material in professional journals related to clergy-perpetrated sexual abuse (CPSA). To further their understanding, the authors, in partnership with other clinicians and religious leaders, conducted a series of half-day focus groups that included survivors and their family members to consider the impact of CPSA. These often emotionally charged groups elicited valuable insights and established a foundation for future collaborative planning with those most directly affected by CPSA and by the scandal. The presence of major symptoms of post-traumatic stress disorder (PTSD) as well as common co-occurring problems, including substance abuse, affective lability, and relational conflicts, was repeatedly confirmed through the personal testimony of survivors and family members. Yet additional themes were also noted, particularly the impact on the family, a profound alteration in individual spirituality, and a change in individual and family religious practices. Following these focus groups, a conference to examine the impact of CPSA with particular attention to family relationships and spirituality was offered in June 2005 in collaboration with the Boston College Church in the 21st Century initiative and the Boston College Graduate School of Social Work.

This special volume, devoted to furthering our understanding of CPSA, was conceived as a result of those powerful conversations and encounters. Two principles governed the selection of articles and authors for this project. First, we believe it is vital that the voices of survivors, their families, and others impacted by these crimes and by this scandal are heard. Second, this volume should advance our understanding of the unique traumatic impact of CPSA.

Part 1 of this volume offers survivor perspectives captured through the qualitative research of Paul Isely and Kathryn Flynn. Dr. Isely's research, originally conducted in 1996, provides one of the first in-depth accounts by nine men on how childhood sexual abuse by Catholic priests impacted them immediately and in the years that followed. Dr. Flynn examines the impact of CPSA on 25 women who were abused either as children or adults. Leslie Wind, James Sullivan, and Daniel Levins conclude this section with a consideration of the impact of CPSA on the family.

Part 2 considers CPSA in the context of religious beliefs and communities. Joseph Guido outlines Catholic theological beliefs and how these beliefs complicate the impact of sexual abuse when the perpetrator is a member of the Catholic clergy. Amy Neustein and Michael Lesher detail a single case of alleged rabbinical sexual abuse and illustrate how Orthodox Jewish beliefs influenced the response to those allegations. Both articles underscore how religious beliefs and traditions and the exercise of religious authority influence survivors' healing. Paul Kline and colleagues continue the discussion by considering the impact of CPSA on the general parish community within the Catholic Church. Together, these articles advance our understanding of the unique impact of abuse by religious figures on the cherished faith traditions and religious practices of victims and faith communities.

Part 3 examines this unique form of betrayal and abuse through the lens of psychosocial theories. A group led by Jason Fogler and based at the National Center for PTSD in Boston opens this section by considering a theoretical context that can be used to further our understanding of CPSA. They draw on existing trauma literature as well as develop theoretical underpinnings that are related to the unique features of CPSA. Additionally, in a second article, Fogler and colleagues consider the role of gender in CPSA, underscoring the importance of understanding the abuse as it fits with the individual's developmental stage. In both articles, the authors acknowledge the need for further empirical research and outline areas ripe for further exploration. Stephen Brady completes the third section by discussing the impact sexual abuse has on gay identity development. Through the use of case material and theory, he illustrates the importance of both a gay man and his therapist understanding sexual identity development.

Part 4 presents interventions that can be applied to CPSA. Douglas Noll and Linda Harvey first place the principles of restorative justice in the overall context of civil and criminal jurisprudence and then explain their application, on both an individual and institutional level, to CPSA. Kenneth Pargament and colleagues considers the spiritual dimension of CPSA, first by showing how an individual's spirituality can be negatively impacted by CPSA, then by providing guidance to clinicians trying to address spirituality in the treatment process.

Together these 11 articles bring together a range of authors with varied backgrounds, including survivors, clergy, mental health professionals, and survivor advocates. We hope this selection of topics and authors gives an authentic voice to the many thousands of individuals who have suffered CPSA and points the direction for effective treatment and further research.

REFERENCE

The John Jay College Research Team. (2004, February 27). *The nature and scope of the problem of sexual abuse of minors by Catholic priests and deacons in the United States: A research study conducted by the John Jay College of Criminal Justice (National Clergy Sex Abuse Report)*. Retrieved June 21, 2008, from www.jjay.cuny.edu/churchstudy/main.asp

SURVIVOR PERSPECTIVES ON THE IMPACT OF CLERGY PERPETRATED SEXUAL ABUSE

In Their Own Voices: A Qualitative Study of Men Abused as Children by Catholic Clergy

Paul J. Isely
Peter Isely
Jim Freiburger
Robert McMackin

The sexual abuse of children by Catholic clergy rose to national attention in 2002 following a series of articles in the *Boston Globe* (Investigative Staff of the Boston Globe, 2002). These articles revealed the extent of sexual abuse perpetrated by priests in the Archdiocese of Boston, yet incidents of clergy-perpetrated sexual abuse had been coming steadily forward for at least 10 years before the *Globe* stories. The pattern of abuse and subsequent cover-up of this abuse by Catholic Church hierarchy, which was noted in Boston, was soon reported in numerous other Catholic Archdioceses within the United States. The *National Clergy Sex Abuse Report* (The John Jay College Research Team, 2004) found that more than 10,667 persons were abused by 4,392 Catholic clergy between 1950 and 2002. The majority of the victims (81%) were boys. As striking as these figures are, it should be remembered they are based on actual reports and do not include incidents of abuse where a formal allegation was not filed. Therefore, the actual number of victims and perpetrator priests may be significantly higher than reported.

Beginning in the early 1990s, litigation in civil cases across the country related to the impact of clergy abuse on male survivors became more common (Geyelin, 1993; Greely, 1993; Kennedy, 1993). At the time of the *National Clergy Sex Abuse Report* in 2004, it was estimated that over $500,000,000 had been paid by the Catholic Church in the United States to settle sex abuse cases. Currently, some estimate the settlement figure to be over a billion dollars (Milligan, 2006). Five Archdioceses (Portland, OR; Spokane, WA; Tucson, AZ; Davenport, IO; and San Diego, CA) have either declared bankruptcy as a result of settlements or experienced serious financial stress related to sexual abuse suits.

While there has been extensive coverage of clergy-perpetrated sexual abuse in the mainstream press, particularly in the past five years, little research exists to assist mental health professionals in their understanding of the unique consequences of this type of trauma (Bottoms, Shaver, Goodman, & Quinn, 1995; Isely & Isely, 1990). The present study was originally conducted by the first author in 1996 as a psychology doctoral thesis at Boston University (Isely, 1996) and remains one of the few qualitative examinations to date of the long-term impact sexual abuse perpetrated on boys by male Catholic clergy. This paper provides a unique window into the experience of men who were abused by Catholic clergy.

The sample will be described in the following sections, followed by considerations of predisposing factors related to abuse. The immediate and long-term impact of the abuse will then be considered along with a discussion including treatment recommendations. The goal of this paper is to give a voice to a small, but we believe representative, sample of the many men who were abused as children by Catholic clergy.

OVERVIEW OF PARTICIPANTS, PERPETRATORS, AND THE ABUSE EXPERIENCE

The nine men in this study were selected in coordination with a nationally recognized advocacy group established for victims of clergy abuse, the Survivors Network of those Abused by Priests (SNAP). All conversations were recorded and transcribed for in-depth analysis. All personal information that would directly identify a subject or perpetrator was removed.

Participants were between 31 and 67 years of age and reported one or more sexual experiences prior to their 16th birthday with an adult male who was an ordained Catholic minister. *Ordained* was defined as the perpetrator having completed the vows for enrollment in a religious order or the priesthood at the time he committed the abuse. All clergy perpetrators were over 18 years old when the offenses were committed and at least five or more years older than their victims.

All participants had some college education and were from middle-class backgrounds. None had a history of sexual victimization prior to their abuse by clergy. Seven men described their home environments as "typically Catholic" and remembered their parents as practicing Catholics (see Wind, Sullivan, & Levins, 2008). Eight of the men described parental relationships as emotionally distant. None, however, reported a history of family mental illness. Only one subject reported having received sex education in school or at home prior to the abuse. Three men reported a nonabusive, age-appropriate sexual experience prior to their sexual abuse by a priest. All but one of the participants had been involved in therapy during their adulthood. Five men had participated in a support group specifically focused on coping with the impact of clergy abuse.

Eight of the perpetrators were described by participants as younger men at the time of the abuse. All were described as having been men in positions of trust: an influential parish priest or high school teacher, for example. All but one was described as having been especially popular with adolescents or younger boys. All of the perpetrators were described as having expressed or demonstrated positive attention to the victims prior to the abuse.

The age of onset of the abuse ranged from 9 to 15 years old. Abuse included fondling, mutual masturbation, and oral sex. Six of the participants reported multiple incidents of victimization. Only one victim disclosed the abuse immediately afterward, while the remaining eight thought they would not be believed or would be punished if they disclosed. Looking back on the experience, all of the men reported having no clear realization that the perpetrators' behavior was "sexual abuse" or of an illegal nature.

FINDINGS

Predisposing Factors Related to Abuse

A theme analysis of the interviews identified several factors present to varying degrees within each victim's life prior to the onset of the sexual abuse that may have served to elevate their risk of abuse. Eight of the parents were practicing Catholics and most victims were active in their local churches as altar boys. Parental reverence for the sanctity and trustworthiness of the clerical state was powerfully transmitted to all participants as children. Therefore, there was little difficulty on the offender's part in gaining access to his victim. Additionally, the need to feel connected with and to receive attention from a father figure and the priest's ability to provide even the slightest fatherly interest to a boy's paternal yearnings was extremely compelling to many. Such adult attention, particularly from a trusted figure of important social status, took on great significance to many of the boys. This intersection of the hunger for adult parental attention and deep regard for the clergy may have made the participants especially vulnerable targets. One subject, abused at 11 years of age, described his father as "never very loving or affectionate." His statement regarding the priest who abused him both speaks to his vulnerability and the emotional need the priest was able to fill in his life at the time.

My parents were always involved in the church. . . . So him and my father, I guess it was like birds of a feather, they just, I guess, clicked. . . . He was very charismatic and all the kids flocked to him and hung out because, ya know, he cussed and drank. It was just like the cool priest . . . Any young Catholic would just flock to someone like that as opposed to the old monsignor. (Isely, 1996, p. 229–230)

Another factor contributing to creating the conditions of victimization concerned the sexual naiveté of the participants at the time the abuse took place. Interviews revealed that, as boys, the victims were remarkably unfamiliar with the reality of sexual abuse. Many reported never having considered the possibility that adults might engage children in sexual activity. Homosexuality was not discussed, although some of the participants remember having been taught that a same-sex relationship was "weird." Participants reported having little to no understanding of male sexuality (e.g., ejaculation or orgasm). This noteworthy innocence or naiveté is revealed in the report of a victim abused over a six year period:

I knew he (the priest) slept with my older brother and when we slept together it kinda clicked to me that he must have been doing this to my older brother, too. And he (the brother) never said anything about it, if it was wrong, so it must be something that could be acceptable. (Isely, 1996, p. 264)

Impact of the Abuse in Childhood and Adolescence

Although the duration of abuse for three of the boys may have included only a single event, all of the victims reported acute disturbances in psychosocial functioning in the immediate aftermath of the initial abusive encounter. All but one reported experiencing intense fear that others would find out what had happened. Seven men reported difficulty remembering portions of the abusive events, and most reported being troubled with some intrusive memories. All reported feelings of low self-esteem and low self-worth. For most, the experience with the priest was their first sexual contact. Most wondered why they were selected, feared that they were somehow attracting men, and five reported questions regarding their sexual identity. A victim who was abused over a three year period gave this account of what took place right after the abuse. His account explains some of the repression of memories that was often reported in childhood post abuse. He stated:

When we got home, I remember running in the house and just running upstairs and locking myself in the bathroom for a long time. When I came out, I could not face my mother and tell her anything about it because I knew it was a very evil thing and could not share it with her. So, I locked that memory in very tight. (Isely, 1996, p. 175)

Immediate difficulties with trust were also pervasive during childhood for most victims after their initial abuse experience. The severe betrayal of trust by the perpetrator combined with the belief that they would not be believed by others produced noteworthy changes in social functioning, including increased periods of isolation from others and few friendships. Many of the subjects attempted to establish peer relationships, but they were often strained, troubled, and emotionally labile. A participant, abused over a two-year period beginning at age 10, described these difficulties with trust:

I mean, if you and I couldn't trust our parish priest; excuse me. Point out someone to me that I can. This is the one guy who came with all the credentials that was certified as trustworthy and we couldn't trust him. Now, what more could you want for a certification of trustworthiness? (Isely, 1996, p. 359)

Participants also reported feeling an immediate burden of personal shame, which for many contributed to problems with destructive anger and rage. Eight of the men recalled intense feelings of shame during and after the abuse, including irrational and deep pervasive guilt for the abuse. One victim who was abused over a seven year period described the link between shame, guilt, and anger:

I took it all on myself. I was a martyr. Psychologically, I'm probably passive aggressive. I turned anger into guilt and then I lashed out in little devious side ways. So my anger for him was growing. It began to grow from that point. And it took four years before I could let it out. (Isely, 1996, p. 314)

For all participants, the complex and immediate reactions to the abuse, shaped, in part, by preexisting psychosocial beliefs and experiences, resulted in the development of a pattern of self-defeating ways of functioning that influenced, in powerful ways, later adolescent development (see Fogler, Shipherd, Clarke, Jensen, & Rowe, 2008). All reported chronic intense inner turmoil. New developmental challenges often proved overwhelming as a consequence of enduring self-blame for causing or failing to prevent the abuse and the associated deep shame. The ongoing development of a meaningful personal identity was further undermined by fear that the abuse was evidence of homosexuality, resulting in continuous pressure to guard the secret of the abuse and a relentless fear that others would find out this secret. Their first sexual contact, within the context of both creating a friendship and/or a surrogate father relationship, appears to have created a synergistic effect within their developing adolescence, rupturing the process of crucial interrelational tasks and inducing a series of emotional disruptions that would persist into their adulthood. Two participants, both abused at 14 years, described the impact of sorting through the complexity of their adolescence as follows:

> Well, I lived in this fantasy world. I don't think I was ever too much in touch with reality. It's [the abuse] taken me away from myself in the sense that I never made choices for me. You know I never did what I wanted to do or really wanted to do . . . I didn't know who I really was. (Isely, 1996, p. 297)

> I felt like an adolescent until I was probably forty. . . . I couldn't get along with my parents. I didn't invest in the trappings of adulthood until I had to. (Isely, 1996, p. 422)

Long-Term Impact of Clergy Abuse

All of the participants experienced intrusive memories, and three reported experiencing flashbacks as adults. Many did not recall feeling depressed or experiencing significant emotional distress before the onset of abuse. All reported symptoms of mood disturbance, such as low self-esteem, poor sleep, suicidal ideation, anger, and detachment from others following the abuse and intensifying in adulthood. All but one reported periods of intense confusion and anger related to the sexual abuse. As adults, seven men continued to experience guilt related to some aspect of the abuse. Expressions of shame were also common (see Fogler, Shipherd, Rowe, Jensen, & Clarke, 2008). Six of the participants had periods as adults where they felt frightened about remembering the abuse and/or confronting the abuser. Three struggled with symptoms of dissociation and two reported this as an ongoing and chronic problem. The following two quotes are from a victim abused in mid-adolescence and speak to the enduring impact of the sexual abuse.

It keeps me isolated. It keeps me from experiencing myself and others on a much deeper level. It keeps it very superficial. It's like a tremendous emptiness, like a desert. But once in a while, you'll come along and there will be an oasis there, and it will be green and alive, but it doesn't last. It's like a mirage. (Isely, 1996, p. 298)

Two years ago my sister died. We were at the funeral parlor and the very first person who walks into the room is him, my perpetrator . . . I was in a near panic. I really was. I wanted to leave the room. I wanted to go hide, but I didn't. My wife made sure I didn't. . . . It's a blur what happened. I asked my wife what did I do? He extended his hand to me and apparently, from what she tells me, I shied away totally and turned away from him. So there was a feeling of panic and fear. (Isely, 1996, p. 182)

Seven of the participants evidenced difficulties in their ability to recall aspects of the abuse with complete clarity, with those abused by multiple perpetrators showing the greatest difficulties. Three of the men, for example, were unable to remember entire periods of their late grade school years. Most described the experience in adulthood of remembering new details of their abuse and reported that fragmented memories still surface. Some have decided not to actively pursue uncovering possibly forgotten events. Seven men reported continuing to experience difficulty constructing an exact chronology of the abuse, stating that their memories were often blended or blurred together. This made it difficult for them to clearly present their abuse as a fully coherent story. All but one of the participants disclosed their abuse only after many years of silence. Four first disclosed to individuals affiliated with counseling or psychological treatment, while four others first disclosed to a relative or friend. Five participants, as adults, reported the abuse to representatives of the Catholic Church. Of those, three described the experience as negative, increasing their distrust of the church. The following quote is taken from a letter a survivor, abused over a four period, wrote to his abuser. Rather than send the letter, he gave it to the Chancellor of the diocese where the abuse occurred. His words speak to the need to disclose that the majority of victims felt as adults.

The time has come at last. I can no longer keep my silence. I must unburden my conscience and rid myself of the horror I have been living with for the greater part of my life since you abused me as a young seminarian. Yes, I remember the occasions and I am sure you do . . . I now know I was completely and totally innocent of any wrong doing. The nagging memories, the dark shadows that lurk in my mind were not my doing, but yours. (Isely, 1996, p. 182)

Participants' testimonies strongly indicated that sexual abuse by a Catholic priest against a pubescent boy acted as a developmental insult with a high likelihood of compromising social, relational, and intrapsychic functioning in later life. If emotional difficulties were present in the child, the negatively based internalized thoughts and reactions to the abuse insidiously integrated themselves within existing difficulties, solidifying and exacerbating them with the negative effects enduring into adulthood. All nine men reported that the sexual abuse impacted negatively on their adulthood and all reported a belief that some part of them was severely damaged by the abuse. It was not uncommon for them to describe themselves as "damaged goods" or to disclose feelings that they somehow harbored a core sense of inner "badness." All of the men reported feelings of low self-esteem and pervasive feelings of inadequacy that extended into adulthood. Another common theme was a deep sadness about how their lives could have been different given another set of circumstances. A participant who had been abused for six years described his sense of feeling damaged and how it impacted him as an adult: "It was kind of like I built a wall around myself and I could look out, but nobody could really see me. I didn't want people to really know me" (Isely, 1996, p. 266).

All but one man described feeling ashamed about the abusive past and, as a result, many of those men believed themselves to be essentially unlovable. As adults, they also believed that people would reject them if they revealed their "true" self. For many, this sense of having a "counterfeit identity" shaped a relational style that was avoidant of other people outside of superficial interactions. All reported spending their adult life feeling estranged from other people and actively avoiding relationships with men. Three men struggled with fearful feelings regarding homosexuals and their own sexual identity. The consequences of this combination of core hateful beliefs about the self and self-defeating patterns of relating to others were most painfully witnessed in participants' descriptions of their romantic relationships and relationships with family. Five men reported a history of promiscuous or compulsive sexual activities. A participant, abused at the age of 13, described the impact his abuse had on his ability to develop healthy relationships:

In every way it had a negative impact. I had no awareness of just how pervasive the negativity was. Basically, trusting and fearing. That's preventing me from having healthy relationships. The one time I did have a healthy relationship with sexuality blended in, and was not threatening and non-scary, it scared the shit out of me. I mean, I look at it now as it was totally different than the behavior that had been modeled and I was modeling. But, when it finally was good, it didn't make any sense to what I was used to and I pushed it away. (Isely, 1996, p. 222)

DISCUSSION

This study described the enduring impact of sexual abuse of boys by male Catholic clergy and raises implications for treatment of victims in adolescence and adulthood. Since male victims tend not to disclose their history of sexual molestation (Dimock, 1988; Finkelhor, 1984), care must be taken in assessing for sexual abuse histories with male clients. Clinicians should not assume that either a child or adult survivor necessarily understands that the sexual contact was sexually abusive. At its initial occurrence, participants in this study did not identify the violence against them as "sexually abusive," and this initial difficulty in naming the experience as abusive may have hampered their ability to effectively cope with the trauma. When they did reach this understanding of abuse much later in their adult years, it appeared to have produced some relief from the complex mix of painful feelings that had remained deeply embedded within them. Helping clients understand that sexual contact between any adult and child is wrong, regardless of the adult's affiliation or status, will assist those who are confused about the responsibility of such experiences.

Participants in this study described sophisticated and effective manipulation by perpetrators to secure their silence, including being told that they were dirty or evil, they invited or caused the perpetrator to have sex with them, they would not be believed by others, they would be punished for what they did, they would be taken from their home, they deserved to be abused, they were "chosen" over others to receive either the abusers or God's "love," they would show love of God by not telling, or they would be hurt if they told. These manipulations cause children to believe that being abused is what they are "good for," and, for others to like them, it is an experience they must accept. Since the priest-perpetrator is seen as a representative of God and a highly revered and respected person in the community, victims are often coerced into believing that being sexually abused is their expected role and the way religion is expressed through them (see Guido, 2008). Rather than feeling the sorrow, rage, pain, and guilt associated with their abuse, many victims develop elaborate defense systems that allow them to cope with the dysfunction occurring in their lives. A dread of impending punishment from God or others can keep victims alienated from religion but also from themselves and loved ones.

Most of the men in this study required extensive therapy in order to effectively address these issues. The course of treatment may last many years. Establishing a safe relationship with an authority figure who offers opportunities for the men to risk intimacy and vulnerability appears to have been an important, critical factor in recovery. Research also suggests that male victims may also require a therapeutic format that provides psychosocial education components to assist in understanding human sexuality and the dynamics involved in sexual perpetration (Bolton, Morris, & MacEachron, 1989; Isely, 1992).

It can be expected that many men will present with features of post-traumatic stress disorder (PTSD), which will require clinicians to understand the nature by which traumatic events interweave themselves into the survivor's life. Based on this study, it is likely that many men will be socially isolated even if they are married and have families. Approaching intimacy is a fearful process, born of mistrust and a need for self-protection. These feelings will probably emerge slowly within the therapeutic environment, demanding a level of careful support. In general, the psychological treatment of adult men who were sexually abused as children by clergy demands a multidimensional clinical approach that can address the various emotional, developmental, and abuse-related phenomena typically seen in survivors of other severe trauma (Bolton et al., 1989).

Given the disruption of the men's ability to trust and nurture relationships with peers and authority figures, therapy is often a gradual process, and ambivalent feelings toward the therapist may frequently arise. Since many of the participants had avoided consciously thinking about both their abusive past and the impact that it has had in their lives, it will be important to carefully assess for depression, suicidality, PTSD, and relationship and sexual dysfunction. Based on their restricted ability to express emotions, it can be expected that nurturing therapeutic environments will allow the surfacing of powerful feelings previously unavailable to them. These emotions, often suppressed for decades, may produce intense fear and avoidance in men who have typically shunned powerful feelings of anger and grief. Assisting them in moderating such feelings will be an important aspect in stabilizing symptoms while maintaining a therapeutic relationship. Such feelings may also be projected onto the therapist who has provided the context and relationship for such emotions to emerge. Since most of the men had not confronted their perpetrators, it is likely that the therapeutic encounter will be a vehicle to experience those emotions. In light of these difficulties, therapists may need to prepare themselves for a variety of experiences that represent unresolved aspects of the male survivor's damaged sense of self.

As indicated by the study, the men's ability to directly address these abusive experiences appeared to reduce the intense symptomatology associated with the onset of their molestations. Their typically avoidant style, however, suggests that this process must be pursued carefully, in a manner in which the client feels free to choose the timing and extent of their disclosures. Therapists who attempt to impose timelines on client disclosures may inadvertently re-create dynamics inherent in the past abuse by defining how these men should think and feel, and at what time.

Based on the findings of this research, interpersonal skills building and the establishment of peer relationships will be an important therapeutic outcome for male survivors. The unique nature of clergy-perpetrated sexual abuse suggests that individual treatment might be successfully augmented by a support group that can both validate and decrease the interpersonal isolation evidenced among survivors.

Eight of the nine men came from families of actively practicing Catholics, yet only three remained marginally involved with their faith as adults. Considering the offenders' affiliation with religion and the central aspect faith played in the lives of most men, it is important for the therapist to pay attention to the effect of the abuse on spiritual beliefs and practice (see Pargament, Murray-Swank, & Mahoney, 2008).

Clergy-perpetrated sexual abuse acted as a developmental insult that arrested many crucial tasks in the participants' psychological maturity, limiting their ability to fully trust themselves and those around them. Although frequently succeeding in establishing families, participants reported feeling detached from their feelings and risked intimacy only within a narrow and impaired context. For most of the men, telling the secret of their abuse and sharing these stories with their families and/or within the therapeutic relationship helped to alleviate or reduce many of the symptoms associated with their abuse. Their participation in support groups and other forms of treatment resulted in validating a seemingly unique type of abuse that had solidified their sense of isolation and mistrust.

Nonetheless, in spite of these complex difficulties, the men in this study evidenced remarkable resilience. Although many of them struggled through an intense period of sexual promiscuity, none of them reported the emergence of deviant sexual predilections. The majority of men married or formed significant love interests. Some of the men had children, as well as positive and loving relationships, and none reported that they had physically or sexually abused children. This resilience can be seen in the words of a 67-year-old survivor, who was abused at the age of 13:

> It has been a long journey, but I feel good about it now. But, there is a terrible feeling of what might have been, if that had not happened to me. If this hadn't happened way back as a kid, I think I would have been much different—much feelings of regret. I feel as if my married life would have been different. My sexual problems would have been less. Yes—much regret. (Isely, 1996, p. 182)

CONCLUSION: VICTIM TO SURVIVOR

Every individual sexually abused by a priest both desires and fears revealing his trauma to others. The desire arises from a need to make meaning from anguish and a wish that it will never happen to other children. The fear is that it will not be remembered or that the experiences will make loved ones uncomfortable, raising difficult, inconvenient, and often unanswerable questions.

To say that the individual can be healed of his abuse wounds is not to say that he can be what he would have been before the abject touch of the abuser entered his body and soul. Healing neither restores one to a previous state nor confers the magical status of the normal. But healing does mean that every abuse victim, no matter what his private pain, can fully assume the human vocation to be happy. Yet for healing to take place, it can never be a happiness that excludes, and certainly never one that forgets.

The journey from victim to survivor begins in a profound betrayal that must be acknowledged for what it is: a sexual assault fostered by manipulation, deception, and deceit, and often perpetrated in the name of God. It is never based in love since real love cannot be seduced, forced, or coerced in any way. Each journey is an individual one with few maps and one not all can make. The sides of the road are lined with casualties, such as the friend of one the authors, a survivor a sexual abuse who shot and killed himself on a past Christmas Eve.

Yet there are fellow travelers, particularly those who share a similar experience. It has been the experience of the authors of this paper that peer support is a critical aspect of any healing.

REFERENCES

Bolton, F. G., Morris, L. A., & MacEachron, A. E. (1989). *Males at risk*. Newbury Park, CA: Sage.

Bottoms, B. L., Shaver, P. R., Goodman, G. S., & Quinn, J. (1995). In the name of God: A profile of religion-related child abuse. *Journal of Social Issues, 51*(2), 85–111.

Dimock, P. T. (1988). Adult males sexually abused as children. *Journal of Interpersonal Violence, 3*(2), 203–221.

Finkelkhor, D. (1984). *Child sexual abuse: New theory and research*. New York: The Free Press.

Fogler, J. M., Shipherd, J. C., Clarke, S., Jensen, J., & Rowe, E. (2008). Impact of clergy-perpetrated sexual abuse: The role of gender, development, and posttraumatic stress. *Journal of Child Sexual Abuse, 17*(3–4), 329–358.

Fogler, J. M., Shipherd, J. C., Rowe, E., Jensen, J., & Clarke, S. (2008). A theoretical foundation for understanding clergy-perpetrated sexual abuse. *Journal of Child Sexual Abuse, 17*(3–4), 301–328.

Geyelin, M. (1993, November 24). The Catholic church struggles with suits over sexual abuse. *Wall Street Journal*, pp. 1, 8.

Greely, A. M. (1993). How serious is the problem of sexual abuse by a clergy? *America. 168*(10), 6–10.

Guido, J. J. (2008). A unique betrayal: Clergy sexual abuse in the context of the Catholic religious tradition. *Journal of Child Sexual Abuse, 17*(3–4), 255–269.

Investigative Staff of the Boston Globe. (2002). *Betrayal: The crisis in the Catholic Church*. Boston: Little, Brown and Company.

Isely, P. J. (1992). A time limited group therapy model for men sexually abused as children. *Group, 16*(4), 233–246.

Isely, P. J. (1996). In their own voices: A qualitative study of men sexually abused as children by Catholic clergy. *Dissertation Abstracts International, 57*, 5328–5329.

Isely, P. J., & Isely, P. (1990). The sexual abuse of male children by church personnel: Intervention and prevention. *Pastoral Psychology, 39*(2), 85–99.

The John Jay College Research Team. (2004, February 27). *The nature and scope of the problem of sexual abuse of minors by Catholic priests and deacons in the United States: A research study conducted by the John Jay College of Criminal Justice (National Clergy Sex Abuse Report)*. Retrieved May 15, 2008, from http://www.jjay.cuny.edu/churchstudy/main.asp.

Kennedy, E. (1993, March 19). The see-no-problem, hear-no-problem, speak-no-problem problem. *National Catholic Reporter*, p. 5, 8.

Milligan, S. (2006). Abuse cost churches nearly $467m in '05. *Boston Globe*. Retrieved March 18, 2007, from http://www.boston.com/news/nation/washington/articles/2006/03/31/abuse_cost_churches_nearly_467m_in_05/

Pargament, K., Murray-Swank, N., & Mahoney, A. (2008). Problem and solution: The spiritual dimension of clergy sexual abuse and its impact on survivors. *Journal of Child Sexual Abuse, 17*(3–4), 397–420.

Wind, L. H., Sullivan, J. M., & Levins, D. J. (2008). Survivors' perspectives on the impact of clergy sexual abuse on families of origin. *Journal of Child Sexual Abuse, 17*(3–4), 238–254.

In Their Own Voices: Women Who Were Sexually Abused by Members of the Clergy

Kathryn A. Flynn

The phenomenon of sexual abuse by clergy uncovered in recent years through the widespread efforts of media, advocacy, legal, and, most important, survivors coming forward has focused largely on men abused as boys. Unfortunately, due to inconsistent and even nonexistent reporting standards among religious institutions regarding clergy-perpetrated sexual abuse (CPSA), the scope of the problem for women has remained minimally assessed. A majority of offenders are male. One major denominational panel reported that "women are more likely to get sexually harassed in the church than in the workplace," and "clergy are sexually exploiting their parishioners at twice the rate of secular therapists" (Grenz & Bell, 1995, p. 22). Additionally, the problem of CPSA of women has too often been normatively misunderstood and believed to be one of sexual ethics rather than professional misconduct. This formulation of the problem often places blame on the entrenched notions of the woman's deviant or seductive character rather than on the aberrant behavior of the offending clergyman.

When describing or explaining any problem, the language used is a powerful cultural and social tool that can influence perception. The language used to explain CPSA of women, including minors, reveals deeply ingrained social attitudes and, coupled with religious leadership's power to name and define, often wrongly describes this abuse as "consensual." At times, this misinterpretation has even been adopted by some female abuse survivors, who, like survivors of incest, often mistakenly believe themselves to be responsible for their abuse regardless of their gender. The Reverend Dr. Marie Fortune was the first to bring national attention to CPSA of women, and with consistent clarity has placed strong emphasis on correctly identifying abuse as a grave violation of a clergyman's professional boundaries. Naming the violence of sexual abuse remains crucial to stopping it. Violence was violence, she has noted, no matter what form it takes (Fortune, 1983, 1988, 1989, 1993, 1995; Fortune & Poling, 1993, 1994). Thus, like rape, CPSA is not an issue of sexuality but rather one of a power imbalance that negates any possibility of "consensual" mutuality. This distorted power dynamic has been accentuated by some clergy abusers through the misuse of significant social, cultural, and even supernatural power ascribed to religious representatives as being derived from God (Bisbing & Jorgenson, 1998; Fortune, 1989; Fortune & Poling, 1994; Francis & Turner, 1995; Grenz & Bell, 1995; Maris & Hopkins, 1993; Milgrom & Schoener, 1987).

Besides the significant power differential, women are impacted by sexism found in the hierarchical structure of many institutional churches and resident in broader cultural norms. This sexism can contribute to an uninformed social definition of these relationships, often defining them as "affairs" and not as occasions of interpersonal violence arising from a disparate power dynamic in which the central defining nucleus is the infliction of harm. Consequently, others, including many victims themselves, have held women responsible for their own exploitation. Women who have been abused by clergy have lacked the communal vocabulary to view the experience as a professional boundary violation of abuse, which includes a component of systemic violence rather than representing a highly personal difficulty (Bergen, 1996). This worldview, which holds women equally or more responsible for the abuse than the clergyman perpetrating the abuse, influences not only how survivors view their abuse but how it is viewed by the community at large. An informed vocabulary, therefore, innately broadens the awareness of sexual exploitation of women in church as a pervasively entrenched social problem.

This article gives voice to the experience of women abused by clergy. A brief overview of trauma is initially presented, followed by a discussion of how trauma was manifested in a sample of women who experienced CPSA as either children or adults. A more complete copy of the study can be found in *The Sexual Abuse of Women by Members of the Clergy* (Flynn, 2003).

TRAUMA OVERVIEW

The definition of trauma used in this study is derived from Herman's (1992) discussion of trauma as an infliction of helplessness in response to overwhelming events that rupture ordinary systems of adaptation. Trauma involves feelings of "intense fear, helplessness, loss of control, and the threat of annihilation" (Herman, 1992, p. 33) Two core responses to traumatic exposure—helplessness and disconnection—are consistent across all populations. Helplessness is created by burdening psychological systems of ordinary adaptation to precipitate a core response of feeling violated, overwhelmed, fragmented, and powerless to either adapt to or change the situation. Disconnection is a relational schism resulting from the violation of basic trust, injuring the individual's connection to others. It is marked by decomposition or disintegration of attachment and relational meaning. Traumatized individuals characteristically feel shattered in identity or strangely unfamiliar to themselves, abandoned, outside systems of care, invisible, silenced, shamed, and alone (Herman, 1992; McFarlane & deGirolamo, 1996; Newman, Kaloupek, Keane, & Terence, 1996; Peterson, Prout, & Schwarz, 1991; van der Kolk, 1996).

In addition to the clinically recognized post-traumatic stress disorder (PTSD) diagnostic criteria of intrusion, hyperarousal, and constriction, Herman (1992) also describes a push-pull dialectic where the individual vacillates between an uncompromising need to deny the occurrence of an event even while simultaneously being subjected to an intensely horrific compulsion to speak the unspeakable and accommodate the event into linguistic and cognitive structures as a hallmark response to traumatic exposure. Individuals experiencing traumatic exposure can endure powerful incongruous symptoms where "the two contradictory responses of intrusion and constriction establish an oscillating rhythm" (Herman, 1992, p. 47). Individuals may fluctuate between the intrusive invasion of repetitive thoughts or flashbacks and the anesthetizing dissociation that shields conscious awareness from these very threatening onslaughts of reexperiencing. For many, to speak or not to speak becomes an invariable, unalleviated, tormenting question. Many struggle to reconstitute a divided self into a single self by dissipating the contradictory aspects of their traumatic response. Often the ability to articulate undifferentiated emotions becomes lost, along with identity and relational capacity. For many, this is "the most characteristic feature of the post-traumatic syndromes" (Herman, 1992, p. 47).

Herman and others believe that the response to trauma resulting from prolonged interpersonal violations may better be understood as a spectrum of conditions rather than a single monolithic disorder as outlined in the *Diagnostic and Statistical Manual of Mental Disorders* (DSM-IV; American Psychiatric Association, 2000). Survivors of repeated interpersonal violation develop complex symptoms that may result in characterological changes beyond the reexperiencing, avoidance, and hyperarousal symptoms associated with the DSM-IV diagnosis of PTSD. These other symptoms, which fit well with Herman's descriptions of helplessness and disconnection, may include: alterations in affect regulation; alterations in concentration, attention, and consciousness; need for personal safety; excessive somatization of physical embodiment of psychological pain; alterations in identity and relational capacity; inability to trust; social isolation; alterations in self-perception involving shame and guilt; preoccupation with the relationship of the perpetrator; and alterations in systems of meaning. Taken together, these symptoms have been referred to as complex PTSD or disorder of extreme stress not otherwise specified (DESNOS; Herman, 1992; Johnson, 1998; Newman, Riggs, & Roth, 1997; Roth, Newman, Pelco-vitz, van der Kolk, & Mandel, 1997). For many women, the trauma of CPSA is frequently protracted, making complex PTSD an appropriate descriptor of their experience.

The remainder of this article will examine the impact of CPSA on 25 women. There are many overlaps among the symptoms or reactions Herman associates with traumatic exposure and the diagnoses of PTSD and complex PTSD. To organize the accounts of the abused women, their experiences will initially be considered as they relate to the symptoms clusters of PTSD and complex PTSD as well as to some of the unique dynamics described by Herman. Second, clergy-specific factors associated with the abuse as well as protective factors will be considered. This format will provide a context for the women to describe in their own words how they were impacted by CPSA.

SAMPLE

There were two inclusion criteria for participants. First, each individual had to be a woman who had been sexually abused by a member of the clergy, and second, she had to provide informed consent to participate. Participants' ages at the time of the interview ranged from 23 years to 68 years, with the mean age for onset of the abuse being 31. Seven women had been abused as minors. All women were from Christian backgrounds. Twenty-four were Caucasian and one was African American. Twenty-four out of 25 participants held a minimum of an undergraduate degree and several had achieved advanced or graduate degrees. The sample consisted of highly educated, mature, intelligent, responsible women with spouses and families. For the majority, their church affiliation was a factor of primary importance, and they had donated significant time to their churches. These women were meaningfully employed in predominately service-oriented careers.

A qualitative research design focusing on data development through the construction of meaning, agency, and consciousness was utilized for the study. The abuse events were intended to be exposed from the perspectives of the participants and then linked to larger sociological constructs through a semi-tructured interview process. In qualitative research, the active voice of the participants must be heard (Acker, Barry, & Esseveld, 1996). Additionally, the researcher herself is considered integral to the qualitative research process. Researcher bias and episte-mological reality contributes to the generation, cultivation, and interpre-tation of the narratives and is a crucial part of the dialectical process of uncovering subjective truth. Researcher bias can be identified but not removed. Nor would deletion of researcher bias be a desirable undertak-ing even if it were possible. Although empirically based, the research design is not intended to be quantitative, clinical, diagnostic, or epidemi-ological. The author's perspective, as she approached the data collection and interpretation, is informed by a background in feminist education and theory.

FINDINGS

PTSD

PTSD screening tools were not administered to participants to deter-mine if formal DSM-IV diagnostic criteria were met. Nonetheless, evidence of PTSD symptoms was noted throughout the interview data and will be presented in the women's words as they relate to the three PTSD symptom clusters: reexperiencing or intrusive thinking, avoidance or constriction, and hyperarousal. Additionally, material related to Herman's (1992) concept of the trauma dialectic will be presented.

Reexperiencing/Intrusion

Reexperiencing may present as an unremitting, relentless interruption that invades, seizes, and possesses anyone whose ordinary adaptation organization has been inundated by memories, thoughts, and feelings associated with the trauma. One participant described this as follows:

> The pain I was experiencing was like cancer pain. It had no meaning. It was endless. There was nothing I could do about it that could bring it relief . . . I couldn't believe that any of this was happening to me. . . . Every waking moment of my time was filled with what was going on in church. That is the truth until this very day. I sat taking my exam. I am studying to be a nurse practitioner. It is very hard work that I am doing in school. I am taking this freakin' exam, and I am thinking about what is going on in my life about clergy sexual abuse. It invades my life all the time. It is always there. I want rest from this. (Flynn, 2003, p. 100)

The repetitious thoughts, nightmares, and invasive flashbacks that significantly impaired an ability to escape replication of the abuse were seen in 17 of the women interviewed. Consequently, these women were often fixated on the traumatic moment, reliving it through recurring intrusions and even duplication of behavioral enactments. They described severe psychological stress from being caught in an endless mesh of symbolic triggers, which caused many of them instantly and repeatedly to relive the abuse, as revealed in the following account.

> But it was like being in hell, you know. To be honest, and, yeah, that's all I could think of. I mean, I was obsessed with this thing. I mean, I could not rid my mind of this man or this—what's going on, you know. It's constantly—I'm constantly spinning my wheels about this thing. It just became my life, you know, for a while. It was really—took over. (Flynn, 2003, p. 101)

This "constant" intrusion of unwanted thinking frequently resulted in a preoccupation with the abuse and was particularly devastating as women were unable to integrate the traumatic experience into existing psychological structures. Trauma reexperiencing can invade and assault an individual. The "taking over" aspect resounded through the reports of 17 women.

Avoidance/Constriction

The narratives of women commonly included descriptions suggestive of avoidance, including "shut down," "wall came up," "shocked," "checked out," "closed off," "couldn't move," and "blocked out." At times, affective constriction included dissociative symptoms, which produced a shield or numbing of overwhelming unbearable affect. For some women, this was a protective mechanism that defended against unbearable painful stimuli as the following young woman's narrative illustrates. Dissociative compartmentalization, or splitting, may lead to the creation of a second self, or "doubling," to assist survival.

> And the actual abuse, what I remember of it, I tend to block a lot of what happened out, so I don't recall everything. . . . And by that point I had blocked so much out of my mind I had no idea what I was saying, if it was real, if this really happened like this, or if I had had a nightmare about it, or, you know—I had gotten to the point where I had actually confused myself about what had really happened . . .

being outside yourself and looking, looking at it happen—yes, watching it happen, being an audience to it, whatever. (Flynn, 2003, p. 95)

When she was abused by her pastor as a young adolescent and unable to physically escape, this participant describes how she removed herself mentally and psychologically from the abusive experience. She watched her pastor's molestation "happen" as a spectator in an audience might. She took flight to a safe place where maltreatment became partitioned in her conscious awareness as unconnected to her. This form of affective constriction or avoidance was seen in 84% of the women interviewed as a means to process the abuse they had experienced.

Hyperarousal

Participants used words such as "jumpy," "jittery," "moody," "on edge really bad," "not able to sleep," "distraught," and "flying off the handle," to describe a heightened level of arousal. Following is one woman's description of the hyper aroused state.

I get very anxious. I can't sit through a church service . . . I guess I had a lot of anxiety attacks . . . I was anxious all the time, which I still fight. . . . I am, most of the time, very anxious and very annoyed easily, just edgy. So I don't know that I've ever found that place because I don't ever feel like I am content . . I've lived so long like this that I don't know what it would be like to be calm or to be completely at peace, if you will, or to be completely relaxed. . . . I cannot imagine that every other person on the planet feels as shaky as this, as nervous as this. . . . And it is irritating because sometimes I would really like to absolutely not feel like . . . my heart's going to jump out of my chest. (Flynn, 2003, p. 90)

Another woman described a similar experience analogous in report from an earlier time in her development.

And I was . . . I would go through periods of time where I wouldn't eat for a couple of days. I just couldn't. My stomach was too nervous. And everyone at school said I was very moody and jumpy and jittery and . . . I remember not being able to sleep, but not the whole night . . . And I had some nightmares. (Flynn, 2003, p. 91)

Both statements describe extreme anxiousness, continuous vigilance, and frequent arousal, which the women associated with the conflicts stemming from CPSA.

Trauma Dialectic

Although not a DSM-IV diagnostic criteria for PTSD, this dilemma has been noted by Herman (1992) and was seen in among 22 of the 25 women interviewed. Many participants provided evidence of experiencing an imperative to tell about the trauma, coexisting with the impossibility of telling. For many this was a dilemma, often compounded by the hierarchical relationship inherent in the abuse and the very real probability that she would not be believed. The following quote illustrates how the isolating and wrenching internal polarization of the trauma dialectic was experienced by many women who believed that the incomprehensible truth was not available to anyone, especially to herself.

> It's wanting to tell because I feel like I'm gagged, and my mouth is gagged, and then other times it's like, oh, shit, I know the repercussions that can happen from trying to tell . . . Maybe somehow this would kind of let up some—let up some of the pressure—because it's like—because there's parts of me that feels like I can't be involved as much as I would like to be. But then there's a lot of anger that I don't want to be involved . . . but I want to be. There's that—kind of like that. Yeah, and I just—it's like—and then I'm thinking, well, if I would tell, I would probably be treated like the rest of the victims—like trash. (Flynn, 2003, p. 104)

Complex PTSD

As previously noted, complex PTSD may typify trauma resulting from persistent interpersonal violation. It can be expressed in subtle symptoms indicative of potentially permanent characterological changes. Symptoms commonly associated with complex PTSD, many of which are similar to Herman's descriptions of helplessness and disconnection, will be discussed. The symptoms of preoccupation with the abuser and alterations in systems of meaning cut across all areas of development and psychosocial functioning and often interfere with the ability to trust, feel safe, concentrate, or form social relationships.

Affect Regulation

Ninety-two percent of participants reported difficulties with affective regulation. They expressed being distressed by their own volatility, not knowing when they might disintegrate. The pervasive emotional lability described by most women can be seen in the following quote.

> My emotions were so mixed because you are angry, and you are hurt . . . You would never know it was coming. I would just freak out. I would just start sobbing, or I would freeze. I couldn't tell him what it was. I couldn't get it out of my mouth because of the same aura that the pastor had over me. I was afraid to say what I felt . . . I would just sob. I don't know how many times I did that. I would sob uncontrollably. (Flynn, 2003, p. 111)

This woman's description of her experiences indicated that she felt that she was unable to manage and moderate her emotions. She expressed feeling of loss of control at moments when she least expected and spoke of her struggle to regain herself. •

A second woman described her devastating loss of control over affective regulation as it related to having power over her own feelings.

> For 20 months I cried. . . . But we had—there were so many losses in that grieving process, we—I found out early on that you just— there's no textbook on step by step how to get through this. . . . I was devastated. I—I considered suicide. I was just—just in a black hole for a long time. . . . Rape. This is a rape. I thought for me it was a soul rape. It was a mind rape. (Flynn, 2003, p. 111)

This woman, as did other participants, characteristically expressed an incomprehensibility of her pastor's abuse and of her immediate and continued difficulty in maintaining affect equilibrium.

Attention Alteration

An alteration of cognitive structures related to an individual's ability to focus, to provide attention, and/or to concentrate is associated with complex PTSD. It takes many shapes and was seem among 68% of the women studied, as can be seen in the experience of the woman quoted below.

> I got up one morning and called my boss and said, "I don't know what is the matter with me? I can't think." I was furious because I couldn't think. I was in a well-respected position in my job. What do you mean, "I can't think"? That is what this thing did for me. It literally took away my ability to speak and literally took away my ability to think. (Flynn, 2003, p. 114)

A second woman described a decreased concentration ability, which she directly attributed to the sexual abuse by her pastor.

> My attention span—I lose it a lot. Like I can't keep my attention on some things for very long. I tend to go somewhere else, if you will . . . not, not like I dissociate, but just, you know, I have a hard time paying attention to things. It—it's—it's just, uh . . . the problems always seemed to be pointing back to that incident, and that's where all my other issues were pointing to. (Flynn, 2003, p. 115)

Need for Personal Safety

Fourteen of the women were concerned that disclosure of the abuse might result in further violation to their personal safety, including emotional, spiritual, psychological, and physical safety. In addition to the wrath of the abuser and other church leaders, many women also faced angry congregations and, sometimes, angry friends and family members. These fears and actual experiences impacted the multidimensional aspects of a woman's impression of safety as seen in this quote.

> I was scared to death . . . I—I felt the church was a safe place. I, too, was in denial that any wrong goes on inside of the church. . . . It has helped me to grow up as a woman in that you—you have to—the world is a big bad place. And even inside the church you have to be more streetwise than I ever was in life. . . . I've never seen it that it wasn't without intentionality. This pastor intentionally targeted me. This same pastor that victimized me selected thin blond women for the most part. He targeted anyone who was vulnerable. This is a case of vulnerability. I was vulnerable. (Flynn, 2003, p. 121)

Participants revealed that some had very good reason for concern regarding their physical safety. Sadly, vehement reactions to them by congregants when they reported the abuse were not uncommon. For some, this included physical threats, which compounded and alienated their ability to feel at ease in the world:

> So no place . . . I couldn't go any place and feel safe. I didn't feel safe in my own home, on the street, in my job. . . . One of the things that one of the so-called advocates said to me initially was "get out of the house" because sexual abuse is very dangerous. . . . But the hang-up phone calls didn't go away. . . . That is when I said, "This feels like stalking." I hadn't really identified the phone calls and the broomsticks as stalking. I now know that that is what they were. . . . I was also going around calling myself "Nancy." (Laughter) I was like, this is insane. I never tried to hide my identity. I felt like a fool . . . nothing felt safe. (Flynn, 2003, p. 120)

Somatization

For some, the psychological impact of CPSA resulted in noteworthy symptoms of physical distress resulting from prolonged interpersonal exploitation. Twenty-two of the women interviewed reported somatic complaints, which they associated to the trauma. One participant discussed her somatic response as follows:

> I lost the sight in my eye, in my left eye, when this was going on . . . and I was so stressed out when I went, you know, I was getting sick because I—I was so stressed out that I couldn't sleep. I couldn't eat. I just felt awful all the time. My immune system must have just been rock bottom . . . and the doctor says, if your—if your immune system is compromised, or if you're under a lot of stress, you're more susceptible to getting the eye disease. And I'm like, oh great, you know. So, anyway, when it was all said and done, I had five laser surgeries on my eye, and, I can't see anything that way. I can see out of the side of my eye. But I can't see anything up in front of it. (Flynn, 2003, p. 117)

Eating disorders were also noted in a number of women, as illustrated in the description of one woman's weight loss: "I got down to 89 pounds . . . I went to work every day, and I don't know how" (Flynn, 2003, p. 117).

Relationship Alteration

Alterations in relational capacity were the most pervasive and the most disturbing consequences identified by the women in this study. All but one of the 25 women described how CPSA injured relationships that were central to their lives and/or how CPSA caused noteworthy impairment in their capacity to develop trusting interpersonal connections with others. The following quote outlines how one woman's relationship with her daughter was severely impacted.

> I lost my daughter as a result. She and I were very close. To me, even though her circumstances weren't the best, she was still like a gift from God, a beautiful, wonderful child who I right now don't see any more. And that's—and that's my greatest loss from all this—is her. That's the part I can't stand, and that's the part that keeps me hurting so badly. . . . He's the one who abandoned her and did all these things and, and you know, we suffered financially for years. We went without so much, because as a single parent support- ing three girls—and he did nothing. But now, for him to come back into the picture, and of course his thing now would be—like he—the first thing he did was buy her a car. . . . In the process, I lost her. (Flynn, 2003, p. 128)

In her narrative regarding the priest-father of her daughter, the woman described a double relational assault. She not only experienced the trauma associated with bearing and raising the priest's child as a single mother, but also expressed her despair at the intrusion on her relationship with her daughter when the priest returned years later to entice the child away with a new car.

Trust Alteration

The betrayal women experienced through exploitation by clergy in positions of power was noted by 19 women as very destructive of their ability to trust others in interpersonal relationships. This had an enduring quality, lasting long after the abuse ended for most women as illustrated in the following quote.

> It still affects me. I don't trust anybody. . . . I don't want to because I don't trust him . . . I don't trust pastors. One time he came up to me and he was talking to me, like this close, I couldn't handle it. What's his motivation? When I watch men, like older men now, they'll say things to me and all that, and I'll just think, what's their motivation? What do they want from me? It's just

different in how I look at people and their intentions. (Flynn, 2003, p. 131)

Social Isolation

All but two women reported no social support network that could accommodate their experiences of CPSA. The lack of a broad social awareness of CPSA, in conjunction with an institutional denial or even blaming of the victim, compounded the isolation many women experienced. Some women who sought help or attempted to publicly name the accused clergyman described being harshly blamed and revictimized by others. Without a social context that upheld the reality of their abuse, these women felt isolated, neglected, and forgotten. This sense of extreme interpersonal isolation can be seen in the next quote.

So, no, I didn't say anything to anybody about this. I talked to myself about it. But there wasn't, there wasn't a cultural context for this . . . but I couldn't tell anybody. And I think I knew. I think I did know why I was conflicted, but there was no—I couldn't tell anybody. And I didn't for years. I didn't say anything to anybody. I think I dropped—I think maybe I dropped hints here and there to people. . . . But this is something that was mostly endured in isolation. I think you'll find out most victims, probably with any kind of abuse, but especially with clergy abuse, it's so, it's isolated. It happens in secret, and the victim continues to live with that secret. (Flynn, 2003, p. 134)

Stigmatization and Contamination

Experiencing social stigmatization and corresponding severe feelings of shame and/or guilt were identified in 19 of the women interviewed. These feeling often intensified after the abuse became public knowledge as can be seen in the following quote.

But another part of it was when I walked into the church everyone stared. You know, everyone would whisper. Everyone was—you know—or shake their head, or, you know, in disbelief, or whatever. And so, I think it's more that uncomfortable feeling that kept me out of church and well—and well, additionally, he was also there as well. (Flynn, 2003, p. 138)

This experience of being socially stigmatized or branded by others resulting in intense feelings of shame and guilt was especially acute after the abuse became public knowledge for women who consequently felt debased and dishonored within their church and local communities (see Fogler, Shipherd, Rowe, Jensen, & Clarke, 2008). Some were removed from committees, verbally attacked, shunned, threatened, and disregarded in other ways. Additionally, before they understood their experiences as abuse, their own feelings of deep shame and guilt branded them internally in self-depreciatory ways that amplified the traumatic impact of being harmed.

Clergy-Specific Factors

The interview data revealed five factors that were particularly related to clergy abuse. These factors, although not unique to CPSA, were experienced by the women in a manner that was strongly influenced by the abuser being a clergyman.

The Antithetical Nature of the Experience

Twenty-three women reported that the relationship was initiated by the clergyman, and most felt they had been "groomed" over a period of time. Evidence of grooming included the language constructions, reasoning, hinting, and nonverbal communication the abuser used to gain trust, win their affection, and establish a close allegiance before making more overt and covert sexual overtures. For many, this was a "crazy making" phenomenon. The damage was made even more complex and devastating because the abuser was an individual who, through multidimensional layers of social and cultural complexity, embodied God. Women experienced inner conflict when the relationship, defined by the clergyman as "good," did not feel good. Also, the personal experiences of these women did not match the cultural mainline views and norms of the clergyman as an expression of good behavior and morals, which significantly added to the conflicts many experienced in trying to reconcile diametrically opposed realities. The intensity of this antithetical experience can be seen in the following passage.

> I guess that to me, this man was God's messenger. He was next to God. And he was, is very charismatic, very manipulative but in a subtle sort of way that if you are not on to him, you wouldn't recognize it. And I didn't until a couple of years ago. When he would talk

about—whatever he talked about from the pulpit like truth and honesty, and you go down the whole line, of course I believed him. So, when he is saying to me in the privacy of my bedroom that he loves me, of course I believed him. (Flynn, 2003, p. 155)

Being Hooked

Seventy-two percent of the participants described feeling captured in the abuse situation. Many women were employed by the congregation led by the pastor, which added to the complications and enhanced the feeling of being trapped. A number of women saw their abuser as using mind-control tactics to promote their compliance and dependency. The following quote shows both extreme isolation and the experience of being arrested.

No. There was no way out. I had, ah, the relationship actually lasted, I would say about three years. There was—I had a death wish for most of those three years. Because I—there was no way out of it. . . . But the death wish was, how, how would this end? . . . I didn't understand, what had gone on in the relationship . . . but I didn't understand this mind control. And he was very practiced, Kathryn. He was no match for me. (Flynn, 2003, p. 166)

Misidentification of the Abuse

Eighty-eight percent of those interviewed reported having misidentified the abuse. Initially, some women harshly blamed themselves for the abuse, including those who were children or young adults when they were violated. They expressed initial feelings of intense guilt, shame, and personal responsibility. Some pastors and church leaders went to great lengths to convince women that it was not abuse but rather a mutual relationship between two consenting adults. This made it difficult for many women to consider the possibility that they were not to blame for their own victimization. Correctly understanding power differentials, hierarchical relationships, and professional boundary requirements of the clergy was essential to gaining an accurate perspective of the abuse experience. That the abuse was often accomplished through charm, persuasion, rationalization, and exploitation of closeness complicated this process. The following quote illustrates the importance of properly identifying the abuse.

The other victims that write to me or call me now say just to put a name on it is so healing. It has so much healing power . . . just to be able to say, "Yes, this is what it was." That was so helpful. (Flynn, 2003, p. 183)

Silence and Denial

All but three women reported some degree of shock and revictimization when they attempted to disclose the exploitative sexual relationship. These disclosures were often met by others with disbelief and even overt blaming of the victim. Many individuals endured the pain of abandonment and systemic denial by their institutional church when they least expected it.

> I felt helpless. That is, when I was still in this thing. When I told, I was a victim. Through all that thing, I was a victim to the perpetrator. Then when I told, the church became the perpetrator. I was a victim to the whole institutional system of the church and how they reacted to it. I was surprised. I really thought that Jon [her husband] would go over there and talk to them, the board that he was a member of, and tell them what happened, and they would go, "My goodness. We have to help you guys." It didn't happen that way . . . didn't happen that way. . .I was shocked. I could not believe it. I have since come to realize that that's the way it is. (Flynn, 2003, p. 192)

For some women, denial took the form of active stonewalling and administrative ploys to negate their complaints. Rather than silence and denial, many women encountered open hostility and were victims of aggressive and shaming tactics to discourage their pursuit of grievances.

> I'm not going to go through the whole business with the ministers and how nasty they were. They would at first be very kind to me and within twenty-four hours, they were telling me to get out. . . . Well, obviously what they were telling me in their words that I was a "sick puppy," and I should go to counseling. I was this disgruntled, whining, complaining, sick bitch woman. I was called every name in the book. I used to make jokes about how many names could you have—all this stuff is going on against me. (Flynn, 2003, p. 193)

Living through this revictimization required enormous personal courage, as can be seen below in the account of a woman who was abused when she was 14 years old:

> The people that were in support of him were more vocal, and it hurt a lot to hear people say that I was the—doing it for money and that, you know, that I was just, you know, like unrequited love, you know, things like that . . . and, you know, to talk about what a good person he is. . . . I was like, God, you people don't know him . . . they were saying this was something of a revenge thing and . . . yes . . . yes—oh, and that's nothing compared with what the bishop said about me. He told this to, to this journalist who was writing a book. He told her that I—he said that I was a Lolita. (Flynn, 2003, p. 195)

It was very difficult if not impossible for most women to pursue accountability of a clergyman within their institutional church because of the systemic ecclesiastical denial that created a lack of context for their abuse. Additionally, no viable formal avenues existed for them to process the abuse and seek redress within most congregations. The experience of not being believed had a profound effect on many of the women interviewed regardless of their age at the time of the abuse. Benign framing of boundary violations by religious leaders often reject basic concepts of clergy professional and fiduciary requirement. The silence, denial, and especially blaming of the victim were exceptionally difficult for women to endure:

> And if I speak very bluntly—bluntly about being raped in my home and molested by my pastor, people don't know what to say sometimes. And I understand that, and yet I think that it needs to be said because they think—it happened to you—but it's not going to happen to me! (Flynn, 2003, p. 200)

Relational Spirituality

This fifth clergy-specific area was experienced by 18 women. They described a shift from a transcendent understanding of God as a powerful force ruling the universe to one that was primarily relationally grounded. Their understanding of God had evolved from an almighty God "up there" to a presence "right here and now" between us. While every narrative reported a reorientation in spirituality in response to their abuse, these women described a shift in spirituality to one inherently and primarily relational and humanly oriented. The central meaning and importance of achieving relational connection became an avenue of spiritual awareness. The following account is of a woman's experience of this spiritual change process.

> But there is something bigger than us that we can connect with. I guess that for me the experience of being abused made it impossible to connect. I lost that. Part of what was lost was that connection. I realized a couple years ago that all the things that gave me healing were things that helped me to reconnect with something or establish a connection. It was the disconnectedness that was so traumatizing. Disconnecting spiritually, mentally, psychologically has ramifications across the board. It's like, if I could connect in each one of those spheres, relationally, all those things, then I could get healing, and I could start feeling better. (Flynn, 2003, p. 178)

This increased emphasis on relational connection acquired major importance to many women after they had been exploited, perhaps in response to the disconnection they had experienced. These women maintained deepened spiritual lives even though they had been harmed by their religious institutions, as the following woman's eloquent description indicates.

> What he did, did nothing to my spiritual journey. But what the church did, totally threw me into theological outer space. I had no respect left for the institutional church. I don't want to ever have any respect left for the institutional church. There was essentially no respect. . . . Theologically, I have a—I think I have a high degree of spirituality. But as far as embracing my former beliefs—I don't. I have a tremendous respect for the interpersonal God and a great belief in the interpersonal God. As far as the external God, the one that sits up there and is all powerful and controls the world—don't think He ever existed—He! But the personal God, the interpersonal God that I understand—and I only understand pieces of it—I think She's wonderful! And so I spend my time connecting with an interpersonal God. (Flynn, 2003, p. 180)

Protective Factors

There were a number of relational protective factors that mitigated the negative impact of the trauma exposure for some women. The impact of the abuse was lessened when social consensus and support included open acknowledgment of the abuse and belief of the woman's experiences. When that validation extended into wider circles, especially to include their own faith communities and family, the effect was positive for the survivor. Being believed created psychological confirmation. Prompt removal of the pastor by responsible church leaders, correctly identifying the problem as the clergyman's abrogation of professional responsibility involving malfeasance, and putting support groups in place during disciplinary processes when individuals sought accountability all helped to lessen devastating residues of traumatic impact. The positive impact of such a response can be seen in the following: "Not only did I reach out; they reached back. They helped to love me through this, to talk me through this, and to do everything that was necessary to get this work done. They are still there" (Flynn, 2003, p. 143).

CONCLUSION

This study offers evidence that those women who survive CPSA experience noteworthy symptoms of psychosocial distress that can lead to long-term and possibly permanent impairment in functioning. These symptoms fit with Herman's (1992) formulation of trauma and included symptoms commonly associated with both PTSD and complex PTSD as well as experiences that appeared clergy-specific.

Additionally, many women felt degraded by the denial of the abuse and/or blaming of the victim by church leaders and institutional church structures in response to victim's efforts to seek help (see Neustein & Lesher, 2008). Uninformed viewpoints promulgated within some churches, which implied consent and mutuality when a clergyperson was sexually involved with a congregant and did not recognize the inherently unequal power relationships, negatively complicated a victim's experience. When women reflected on clergy abuse from a vantage point of safety, many identified various forms of manipulation, coercion, and "grooming" behaviors embedded in the relationship and power differentials invalidated any conception of mutuality or consent.

The "abuse" paradigm within churches must be expanded to incorporate adult women. Women's trauma resulting from interpersonal harm needs to be acknowledged and clearly identified. The creation of a context for their experiences is pivotal to ending this largely unrecognized form of human rights infringement. Extensive efforts to create a social context and validation of adult women's experiences within organized religion remain critical. Efforts at a systematic deconstruction of sexist language, including those descriptors that ignore power differentials and portray consent, would be a needed first step. Additionally, every effort both within and outside of organized religion must be made to ensure that women who are sexually abused by members of the clergy do not remain forgotten.

An intriguing finding of this study was the shift among many women toward a relational spirituality in lieu of a hierarchical spirituality dependent on an organized church structure. For the women who made this shift, making a divine/human distinction was essential to bridging the soul wound they described. The current structure of institutionalized religion was unable to meet the needs of many, and they sought renewed spiritual strength through the love of family and friends and regained relational capacity. For them God was found, again and again, through human connection. For these women, divine love had a human face. This inner transformation fits with feminist theory on the importance of relationships within the lives of women and deserves further study.

REFERENCES

Acker, J., Barry, K., & Esseveld, J. (1996). Objectivity and truth. In H. Gottfried (Ed.), *Feminism and social change* (pp. 60–87). Chicago, IL: University of Illinois Press.

American Psychiatric Association. (2000). *Diagnostic and statistical manual of mental disorders* (4th ed., text rev.). Washington, DC: Author.

Bergen, R. K. (1996). *Wife rape: Understanding the response of survivors and service providers.* Thousand Oaks, CA: Sage Publications.

Bisbing, S. B., & Jorgenson, L. M. (1998). *Sexual abuse by professionals: A legal guide. 1998 cumulative supplement.* Charlottesville, VA: Lexis Law Publishing.

Flynn, K. (2003). *The sexual abuse of women by members of the clergy.* Jefferson, NC: McFarland & Company.

Fogler, J. M., Shipherd, J. C., Rowe, E., Jensen, J., & Clarke, S. (2008). A theoretical foundation for understanding clergy-perpetrated sexual abuse. *Journal of Child Sexual Abuse, 17*(3–4), 301–328.

Fortune, M. M. (1983). *Sexual violence: The unmentionable sin.* Cleveland, OH: The Pilgrim Press.

Fortune, M. M. (1988). Forgiveness: The last step. In A. L. Horton & J. A. Williamson (Eds.), *Abuse and religion: When praying isn't enough* (pp. 215–220). Lexington, MA: D. D. Heath and Company.

Fortune, M. M. (1989). *Is nothing sacred?* San Francisco: Harper.

Fortune, M. M. (1993). The nature of abuse. *Pastoral Psychology, 41*(5), 275–287.

Fortune, M. M. (1995). Is nothing sacred? When sex invades the partoral relationship. In J. C. Gonsiorek (Ed.), *Breach of trust: Sexual exploitation by healthcare professionals and clergy* (pp. 29–40). Thousand Oaks, CA: Sage Publications.

Fortune, M. M., & Poling, J. N. (1993). Calling to accountability: The church's response to abusers. In R. J. Wicks & R. D. Parsons (Eds.), *Clinical handbook of pastoral counseling. Studies in pastoral psychology, theology, and spirituality* (Vol. 2, pp. 489–505). New York: Paulist Press.

Fortune, M. M., & Poling, J. N. (1994). *Sexual abuse by clergy: A crisis for the church.* Decatur, GA: Journal of Pastoral Care Publications.

Francis, P. C., & Turner, N. R. (1995, April). Sexual misconduct within the Christian Church: Who are the perpetrators and those they victimize? *Counseling and Values, 39*, 218–227.

Grenz, S. J., & Bell, R. D. (1995). *Betrayal of trust.* Downers Grove, IL: InterVarsity Press.

Herman, J. (1992). *Trauma and recovery.* New York: Basic Books.

Johnson, K. (1998). *Trauma in the lives of children: Crisis and stress management techniques for counselors, teachers, and other professionals* (2nd ed.). Alameda, CA: Hunter House.

Maris, M. E., & Hopkins, N. M. (1993). The victim/survivor. In N. M. Hopkins (Ed.), *Clergy sexual misconduct: A systems perspective* (Special Papers and Research Reports series.) Washington, DC: The Alban Institute.

McFarlane, A., & deGirolamo, G. (1996). The nature of traumatic stressors and the epidemology of posttraumatic reactions. In B. van der Kolk, A. McFarlane, & L. Weisaeth (Eds.), *Traumatic stress: The effects of overwhelming experiences on mind, body and society* (pp. 129–154). New York: Guilford Press.

Milgrom, J. H., & Schoener, G. R. (1987). Responding to clients who have been sexually exploited by counselors, therapists, and clergy. In M. D. Pellauer, B. Chester, & J. A. Boyajian (Eds.), *Sexual assault and abuse: A handbook for clergy and religious professionals* (pp. 209–218). San Francisco: Harper & Row.

Neustein, A., & Lesher, M. (2008). A single-case study of rabbinic sexual abuse in the orthodox Jewish community. *Journal of Child Sexual Abuse, 17*(3–4), 270–289.

Newman, E., Kaloupek, D., Keane, G., & Terence, M. (1996). Assessment of post-traumatic stress disorder in clinical and research settings. In B. A. van der Kolk, A. McFarlane, & L. Weisaeth (Eds.), *Traumatic stress: The effects of overwhelming experience on mind, body and society* (pp. 279–302). New York: Guilford Press.

Newman, E., Riggs, D. S., & Roth, S. (1997). Thematic resolution, PTSD, and complex PTSD: The relationship between meaning and trauma-related diagnoses. *Journal of Traumatic Stress, 10*(2), 197–213.

Peterson, K. C., Prout, M. F., & Schwarz, R. A. (1991). *Post-traumatic stress disorder: A clinician's guide.* New York: Plenum Press.

Roth, S., Newman, E., Pelcovitz, D., van der Kolk, B., & Mandel, F. (1997). Complex PTSD in victims exposed to sexual and physical abuse: Results from the DSM-IV field trial for post-traumatic stress disorder. *Journal of Traumatic Stress, 10*(4), 539–555.

van der Kolk, B. (1996). Trauma and memory. In B. van der Kolk, A. McFarlane, & L. Weisaeth (Eds.), *Traumatic stress: The effects of overwhelming experience on mind, body and society* (pp. 279–302). New York: Guilford Press.

Survivors' Perspectives on the Impact of Clergy Sexual Abuse on Families of Origin

Leslie H. Wind
James M. Sullivan
Daniel J. Levins

INTRODUCTION

The prevalence of clergy-perpetrated sexual abuse (CPSA) rose to public attention in 2002 through the disclosure of a pattern of abuse by Catholic priests within the Archdiocese of Boston and a simultaneous cover-up by church hierarchy. At the initiation of the American Catholic Bishops, a study documented that more than 4,000 priests were accused of some type of sexual misconduct with youth between 1950 and 2002 (National Clergy Sex Abuse Report, 2004). The vast majority (81%) of the more than 10,000 victims noted in the report were boys. While the primary focus of press reports has been on abuse within the Catholic Church, patterns of abuse have also been reported in other Christian denominations (Disch & Avery, 2001; Fortune, 1989).

This article is developed through collaboration between an academic professional and two survivors of CPSA. The Trauma Transmission Model (Figley, 1998) and the Family Adjustment and Adaptation Response Model (McCubbin, Thompson, Thompson, Elver, & McCubbin, 1998) are used to consider the impact of this most intimate, spiritual, and human betrayal on the families of origin of survivors of CPSA. Additionally, issues of reconciliation and healing after such abuse are considered through Figley's Empowerment Model (Figley, 1998). We have drawn on the experiences of the two coauthors with histories of CPSA as well as the limited published survivor accounts to illustrate key points. This paper should be considered exploratory in its examination of such a complex issue as it is based on limited data. The hypotheses and clinical observations offered in this work will need to be reexamined as new data is produced through future research.

The literature on clergy sexual abuse victims and their families of origin, while limited, indicates that many victims of CPSA are individuals whose families were devout believers in their faith (Bera, 1995; Isely, 1996). For example, victims include the children of parish counselors, ministers, master catechists, and volunteers at church functions (Burkett & Burni, 1993). Within many devout Christian family systems, the influence and power of the church and its representatives is pervasive, with an absolute trust given to the individuals and organizations that represent God (Bera, 1995). Daily activities, education, roles, and family identities are deeply intertwined with their religious system and faith. It is through their relationship with their church that many of the families receive emotional, financial, and spiritual support. It was within this context of pastoral care that many children were groomed and then violated. This context potentiated the violation of trust leading to the insult to the family's organizational core, their sense of a faith-based family identity.

FAMILY ADAPTATION TO CRISIS

All traumas have the power to put stress on the family system, interrupt routines, require abrupt changes, and create anxiety. Based on systemic theory, following traumatic exposure all members of the family undergo some level of change (Turnbull & McFarlane, 1996). Communication patterns, role relationships, expectations for behavior, trust that others will meet one another's needs, and flexibility in tolerating differing individual needs can be impacted in a crisis. The traumatic experience, such as child sexual abuse, reverberates throughout the family system (Figley, 1998).

Theoretical Underpinnings

The Family Adjustment and Adaptation Response (FAAR) model (McCubbin et al., 1998) is a family stress model that incorporates coping via alteration of the meaning of a crisis situation. Several theoretical constructs within the FAAR model are central to understanding family adaptation to a crisis such as CPSA. According to this model, a family's *schema* is the organizing structure of shared values, beliefs about the world, and goals and expectations. It is this framework through which the family evaluates crises and legitimizes family patterns of functioning, including any changes. A central function of the family schema is development of family meanings accomplished via appraisal of a crisis situation according to the family's shared values and expectations, shared beliefs, the present and long-term consequences of a situation, and perceptions of personal relationships and interpersonal order in the world. Family *sense of coherence* refers to a family's view about the world being structured and predictable, manageable (via available resources to respond to life demands), and meaningful (Antonovsky, 1987). This construct has been translated as the family capacity for knowing when to enact control and when to trust or believe in the authority of others

(Patterson & Garwick, 1998). Family *paradigms*, or shared beliefs and expectations, guide specific patterns of functioning in relation to family life domains (e.g., communication, spiritual/religious orientation). The family's response to a crisis, then, will be influenced by each of these constructs as they combine to create the meaning the family attaches to the situation (McCubbin et al., 1998).

Two levels of meaning are differentiated within the FAAR model: situational meanings and global meanings. Situational meanings refer to the family's personal definition of the stress demands as well as their coping capabilities and the interaction between them. Global meanings are defined as more stable beliefs about family member relationships and the relationship between the family and larger community (Patterson & Garwick, 1998). Patterson and Garwick present five dimensions of global family meanings, including: (a) shared purpose—family values, goals, commitments; family identity; (b) collectivity—recognizing the family as part of something larger; (c) frameability—viewing situations optimistically and realistically; (d) relativism—viewing life within the context of the current situation; and (e) shared control—a balance of individual and family control with trust in others. They propose that families construct and share meanings on three levels: (a) the specific crisis situation, (b) within the family's identity, and (c) the family's worldview. The situational meaning is determined through communication about the stressor as well as ability to manage the situation. Family identity is reflected in both family membership structure and relational patterns. It is maintained through rituals and routines as well as shared rules and attitudes that organize a sense of the collective. The family worldview focuses on interpretation of reality, core assumptions about the environment, and existential beliefs about the family's purpose and place in life. The view of the family system is shaped by the larger context in which it is embedded. As family members are confronted with a crisis, such as disclosure of CPSA, these constructs influence family dynamics as they negotiate adaptation.

According to Figley (1998), following disclosure of trauma family functioning will adjust in numerous ways to the changes within and between family members. Generally, those in a cohesive family system are likely to draw closer together and search for ways to meet the altered needs of its members. However, families within less cohesive systems with poorer quality attachment become fragmented, with members feeling isolated and unable to experience the closeness and familial trust they desire and need. Communication lines may become blocked, and resentments can develop that are difficult to overcome. Frequently a crisis will also bring long-standing conflicts into the open, often in a dramatic way. Because of how faith may play a supportive and cohesive role in family functioning, when the perpetrator of the trauma is a representative of the family's faith (e.g. a priest) the impact on the family system may be more profound, shattering the family schema, sense of coherence, family paradigms, and ultimately affecting the core identity of the family and its worldview.

Model of Trauma Transmission

Figley (1998) provides a three-stage model of adjustment following trauma disclosure, which can provide a theoretical framework to understand the profound impact of CPSA on a family system. Survivors' quotes are used to illustrate the impact.

Recoil

During this time, some family members may feel very close, experiencing increased intimacy, trust, and communication while long-standing conflicts may be temporarily set aside. At this initial stage of adaptation in families that have experienced CPSA, family members' collective set of core beliefs, including beliefs about the church, the role and status of clergy, and sexual abuse itself (which varies by culture), will influence situational appraisal and the family's coping response.

For many families traumatized by CPSA, the recoil stage is complicated by the fact that survivors waited years before disclosing their traumas. This delay in disclosure, particularly for Catholics, has likely been related to family beliefs about the status of clergy. For example, clergy are somewhat deified, as they are considered God's representative (Knight, 2003). As a result, victimized children have had to struggle with being in a terrible trap, as shared by one survivor coauthor:

> My parents were taught that the Catholic Church, specifically its bishops, priests, etc., was all good and infallible—never to be questioned or doubted. . . . It [disclosure] meant confronting powers greater than me: my parents with their beliefs, the church with its teachings and personnel, and even the town with its rumor mills.

Such theological precepts that ultimately become a part of the family schema and worldview may contribute to family members' disbelief and even blaming the survivor for the abuse when it is eventually disclosed.

The family's worldview, particularly its assumptions about how the church operates as an organizing framework in their lives, is suddenly challenged. Global meanings related to collectivity (e.g., membership in the church), frameability (e.g., capacity to see the future as hopeful), and shared control (e.g., trust in the church) are brought into question. The effect of delayed disclosure can be seen in the words of one survivor who disclosed his abuse almost 20 years after victimization took place.

> Before I came out, my dad would make statements like, "Aw, those victims; someday they are just going to wish they never come forward. They're doing it just for the money. They should keep their mouths shut." I had to listen to all of that. It was painful. After I came forward, I don't think he said a word to me about it. (Isely, 1996, p. 260)

Reorganization

According to Figley (1998), following some stabilization old patterns of communication and old conflicts/role relationships are likely to reemerge, including increased polarization, differentiation, and fragmentation. Such polarization among families impacted by trauma may significantly increase the disconnection among family members, hindering their ability to discuss the trauma. The quality of reorganization will be based on the previous attachment quality of family members and the quality of communication within the family system as well as the resources available to them. According to McCubbin and colleagues (1998), when faced with adversity (such as CPSA), changes in family functioning and the family schema, sense of coherence, family paradigms, and situational appraisal guide the family's response to a crisis. As the survivor's disclosure settles into the family's awareness and there is an appraisal of a need for change in patterns of functioning, family roles may be reexamined and adjusted. In addition, family paradigms, particularly those regarding communication and spirituality and religious orientation, will be confronted and questioned, thereby leading to the emergence of new paradigms that ideally would support changes in patterns of functioning that enhance stability and predictability. In families with good communication skills and a strong sense of coherence that can support alteration of family paradigms, effective problem-solving efforts are more likely available to address the survivor's needs as well as those of the family overall. However, some families will cling more rigidly to their worldview, family schema, and established paradigms. In these families, relationships may be splintered, causing greater distress among family members. For example, continued engagement in roles and routines related to the church where a survivor was victimized could create painful relational divides. One survivor stated how difficult it was to talk about the abuse with his brother, who he believed was victimized by the same priest: "He didn't want to talk about it. He said what was in the past needs to stay there. . . . For me it created a great distance between us" (Isely, 1996, p. 275).

It is during this time that the response of the extended family system, the church officials and congregation, and other sources of social support become tremendously influential in supporting the family's ability to integrate the reality of the trauma. A strong support network will contribute to the family's ability to move into positive restabilization. It should be remembered that in families where a core of their collective identity is invested in their faith community, the reorganization process would be quite complicated. As a family struggles with the legal versus ethical and pastoral response they receive from their faith community, they may experience an exacerbated sense of isolation and traumatic betrayal (Farrell & Taylor, 2000). Altered family schemas, paradigms, and sense of coherence may result in a damaged sense of family spiritual identity (see Fogler, Shipherd, Clarke, Jensen, & Rowe, 2008, for additional discussion of this point).

Restabilization

According to Figley (1998), in the last stage of adaptation family members may try to rebuild their relationships with one another as they were before disclosure. If unable to do so, the family will likely settle into a new period of stability characterized by either deteriorated or increased levels of intimacy, affection, communication, and trust. This restabilization process is often not fully successful, as can be seen in the words of the survivor:

> I guess they [my parents] knew something was up; so, I told them. They believed me. She [my mother] was shocked. She started thinking back on all the things and I guess it clicked together for her. He [my father] never said much. (Isely, 1996, p. 271)

The family response to disclosure will have an enormous impact on the quality of restabilization. As members of the family individually appraise the situation and struggle to synthesize it with both their family schema and their collective worldview, they may experience a secondary traumatic stress response.

SECONDARY TRAUMATIC STRESS IN FAMILIES

As a part of the process of adapting to knowledge of the traumatic experience of a loved one, many family members can experience a range of symptoms similar to those of the direct victims, a pattern often referred to as *secondary trauma* (Manion et al., 1996). There is limited research addressing the issues associated with the secondary traumatic stress of parents and other family members of sexual abuse survivors and no research to date related to families of survivors of CPSA. We will consider secondary trauma first from Figley's (1992) Trauma Transmission Model and then discuss particular familial relationships.

According to the Trauma Transmission Model, many family members are motivated to express empathy for the survivor of the abuse. These family members will attempt to determine what happened, why it happened, the reasons for their own behavior at the time of abuse and since the abuse, and their ability to cope. As a result of the processing of these concerns, they are likely to experience emotions that are similar to those of the survivor, including overwhelming visual images, sleep disturbance, and mood lability. The model suggests that exposure to the stress experienced by the survivor combined with the capacity to experience the feelings of the survivor and a desire to provide support will then determine the empathic response. Two factors are identified as contributing to compassion stress in family members. These include the sense of achievement, or satisfaction, with efforts to comfort the survivor and the degree of disconnection from the survivor, a letting go of the pain associated with caring. Family members who experience less compassion stress due to their ability to let go and who have a strong capacity for empathy are more likely to gain satisfaction from their efforts to care and to experience less family disruption. Families who experience an ongoing sense of responsibility for the suffering caused as well as care of the trauma survivor may be unable to reduce compassion stress and, subsequently, may experience burnout. In such families, there is a likelihood of heightened conflict, disruption, and even separation. Figley (1989) has concluded that families who recognize the individual and family strengths resulting from their struggle to adapt following disclosure of the trauma demonstrate greater recovery.

Building on Figley's (1992) Trauma Transmission Model, within families where there has been CPSA we identify an additional factor that frequently complicates the family's response to the original trauma, which we term *postdisclosure traumatization.* Postdisclosure traumatization here refers to repeated traumatic exposure of survivors and their families through media coverage of the clergy abuse scandal and the church community response. We consider this concept important to understanding the long-term impact of CPSA on survivors and their families who have been repeatedly exposed to stories coming from other churches and dioceses, which replicate their traumatic experience. The impact of this reexposure can further complicate the restabilization process.

Parent-Adult Child Relationship

Following disclosure of trauma, parents often experience a need to reduce their sense of helplessness and will search for ways to explain what happened. Many suffer guilt and anguish about how they might have prevented the abuse. Some families may be a resource for the survivor, and others may become reorganized in a negative manner around the trauma, thereby creating obstacles to healing (Goff & Schwerdtfeger, 2004). While some family members might experience an ongoing closeness with one another, for others the betrayal by clergy could challenge their sense of coherence and leave them feeling inadequate, powerless, and unable to trust their own judgment or trust others.

Sadly, rather than an empathic response to disclosure, a number of victims of CPSA have indicated that their parents' first and sometimes only response to disclosure was disbelief or even self-focused concern. Rather than a concern for the needs of the victim, such family members remained self-protective, utilizing denial and communication patterns that can exacerbate a victim's shame and isolation, perpetuating the secrecy within the family. One such self-protective response was noted by a survivor coauthor, who saw his disclosure as threatening his parents' core belief system and religious identity:

> When I finally had the courage to talk to my parents about my abuse they focused on their own sense of betrayal by the abusing priest who had become a part of our family and the Church. I was taken aback to repeatedly hear, "We didn't know. How dare they do this to us!?"

Sibling Relationships

Siblings of those traumatized may also experience guilt, fear, anxiety, and other traumatic stress symptoms (Applebaum & Burns, 1991; Monahon, 1993). Following disclosure, parents may be so focused on the victim and their needs that they pay less attention to others in the family (Applebaum & Burns, 1991; Matsakis, 2004). Siblings may resent the attention given to the victim, distancing themselves from their sister or brother and parents or acting out their need for support in inappropriate ways. They may blame the victim for the family's distress, become extremely protective, and/or feel guilty about feelings of jealousy (Matsakis, 2004). One coauthor described the impact his disclosure had on a sibling relationship:

> My oldest brother was extremely angry that I came forward to tell my story. He expressed his outrage by demanding to know, "Why are you hurting our parents this way?" He directed me "to keep your mouth shut and get over it!" To this day, my brother will barely acknowledge my existence and when he does a discussion about my abuse and our other brother's abuse is off limits.

Parents' Relationships

Little is written about the impact of child sexual assault on the parental relationship. However, both parents may experience secondary traumatic stress as a result of the trauma of their child. In cases of a child's rape, parental strain can lead to blaming and a lack of support (Hertz & Lerer, 1981). This can be particularly true in families where the clergy perpetrator has endeared himself to the victim's family. When the abuse becomes known, even after a protracted period of time, the parents can feel as if they colluded with the abuser. How this could happen can be seen in the words of one survivor who was abused over a three-year period by a parish priest:

> My mother was a very good cook and as a result, we had a lot of priests around the house all the time. . . . He [the perpetrator] took it upon himself to take us under his wing, so to speak, to keep us in line and showed a lot of interest in us. (Isely, 1996, p. 172)

In a process referred to as resonating grief (Cornwell, Nurcombe, & Stevens, 1977), partners are not only impacted individually but react to one another's distress. Some parents find that talking about the sexual abuse creates enormous discomfort. They may be at odds and define one another's responses as over- or underreacting. Parents are often unwilling to acknowledge the extent of the emotional distress they are experiencing for fear it might lead to a more serious breakdown in family coping. Resonating secondary traumatic stress symptoms can then result in further isolation, avoidance, and denial, thereby increasing family stress (Gilbert, 1998).

Impact on Religious Practices

The betrayal of religious-based trust can create faith-based dilemmas within a family. For example, families may question the holiness of various sacramental rites of passage within the church (e.g., baptism, confirmation, marriage), wondering if previous celebrations were indeed sanctified as they once thought. They may question God's plan for them, wondering why the abuse happened and what it means (Bera, 1995).

A central characteristic of a devoutly believing family is its engagement in daily activities and roles that are wholly intertwined with their religious system (i.e., family paradigms). For such families, there is an individual and a family identity as well as status associated with having significant roles within the church. On a daily basis as well as on a larger scale, families impacted by CPSA may experience a loss of structure related to routine religious practices that previously supported cohesion within both the individual and the family system. For example, after disclosure some members of a family may attend church regularly while others attend sporadically or not at all. For some individuals, attendance may only now be related to a need for the Eucharist. Some may experience a loss of trust in the church of their youth, choosing to no longer share their time and talents with the church. Others may continue to attend church as a family, but parents may not allow their children to be altar servers or do anything that involves the clergy. The effect on religious practices of CPSA for one survivor, who was an alter boy raised in a devout family and abused for two years beginning at age 10, can be seen in the following:

> Father Mike convinced me by his behavior that I know there is no God, because he wouldn't exist. He would not have existed if there was one. I remember I was saying this whole thing is stupid. I used to laugh at people, watching them go to church, putting money in and doing crap. And, I'm thinking these people are idiots. (Isely, 1996, p. 351)

Such strong sentiments expressed within a devout family would likely cause great distress. The threat to their child's religious identity could create a sense of both fear and loss in some parents. They might fear that their child will never regain his/her trust in God and that they would discard their religious identity. They might also experience a loss of their family's religious identity. Among those with a strong faith-based family schema and related family paradigm, such mourning by survivor parents, noted frequently by the survivor authors in their work with other survivors, may be experienced as a traumatic aftershock similar to that experienced by survivors' mourning the loss of their own spirituality (see Kline, McMackin & Lezotte, 2008, for additional discussion).

The assault of CPSA on families' identity and worldview presents numerous challenges for reconciliation and healing. No longer does the family feel secure in its view of the world as ordered, predictable, manageable, and guided by church tradition. No longer can the family engage the same way in daily church-related roles and routines that have provided a sense of organization and a valued place within the world. No longer can the family trust the very community they need for support and understanding during such a crisis.

RECONCILIATION AND HEALING

In spite of the numerous challenges, many families do focus on healing and reconciliation and remain hopeful as they forge changes in family identity, relationships, and their worldview. Figley's (1989) Empowerment Model offers a five-phase approach to mediating the healing process. The five phases include: (a) building commitment to therapeutic objectives, (b) framing the problem, (c) reframing the problem, (d) developing a healing theory, and (e) closure and preparedness. Figley (1998) identified seven goals related to the five phases of intervention, including: (a) clarifying the therapist's role, (b) eliminating the unwanted consequences of trauma, (c) building family social supportiveness, (d) developing new rules and skills of family communication, (e) promoting self-disclosure, (f) recapitulating traumatic events, and (g) building a family healing theory. Successful achievement of these goals requires a sincere commitment to the healing process and the use of honest, thoughtful dialogue by clinician, survivor, and their family throughout the process.

To accomplish these goals, the first three phases of the Empowerment Model focus on creating a therapeutic structure that includes a strong treatment alliance with clarification of client objectives as well as examining how the family perceives the impact of CPSA in their family. Figley (1989) emphasizes the importance of building a commitment to the therapeutic objectives to address such a mutual challenge. Regardless of who decides to initiate reconciliation, when a survivor and his or her family consider addressing the topic of the survivor's sexual abuse by clergy, it is critical to determine each family member's goals. In addition, distinguishing between willingness and readiness to have a discussion within a family system not considered to have been safe enough to expose the sexual abuse when it occurred is a consideration that needs to be addressed. Assuring readiness and willingness, as well as clarifying therapeutic objectives, are key aspects necessary to begin the healing process. Clarification of family members' goals with a commitment to the treatment process, which focus on promotion of positive communication, understanding, acceptance, and a reframing of symptomatic behaviors, often requires a stepping away from blame and a letting go of the anger by both survivor and their family members. In order to do so, at the very least family members need psychoeducation about the dynamics involved in CPSA, clarification about clergy being responsible for the trauma to the child, and ways in which families can assist the adult victim.

Next, Figley's (1989) model of intervention emphasizes a communication process aimed at developing a healing theory. Included in this process are opportunities for family storytelling, a reinterpretation of symptoms, a clarification of insights and correction of distortions, and answers to questions central to healing (e.g., what happened, why did it happen, why did family members act as they did, why have members of the family reacted as they have since the trauma, and how will they cope in the future?). The family can then be assisted in reframing their experiences into a healing story. This communication process embedded throughout the Empowerment Model clarifies the propositions, principles, and assumptions about the CPSA, providing the basis for a family's sense of accomplishment, closure, and the process of reconciliation. This method, then, assists families in reshaping global family meanings related to CPSA, including development of a new worldview, family schema, and family paradigms that nurture reconnection and healing.

When working with individuals and families who have experienced any number of traumas, language is most effective when brought to bear in a positive and supportive manner. Language is not an all-or-nothing proposition; neither is forgiveness nor reconciliation. Both can occur slowly over time. Trauma survivors who have experienced CPSA are likely to be hypersensitive to many environmental stimuli, not the least of which is people's use of language and tone. Our emphasis on the centrality of language in the healing process clearly fits with Figley's (1989) model and its strong focus on communication and information processing. It is language that communicates either overtly or covertly how we feel and what we think. Language, from a CPSA survivor's vantage point, may be two-sided. In considering his own healing, a coauthor describes his experience of the dual nature of language in the following way: "It can be a musical instrument of joy, lighting the darkness that permeates a survivor's very being, or a silent killer, hiding the truth behind unspoken thoughts."

While language can offer hope in the healing process, it may also profoundly exacerbate the trauma, particularly when the abuse is carried out in God's name. For language to be healing, it needs to be reordered and reimagined away from the world of retriggering and into a world where siblings, parents, and others engage in conversations of acceptance of the abuse and its ongoing consequences. When a survivor, even as an adult, enters the disclosure process to develop a healing story, he or she often must address the fears of judgment, further isolation, and/or rejection from those hearing their story (Herman, 1997). This may also be true for parents who want forgiveness from their child. Yet, while those fears may be present Herman reminds us, "healing can only take place within the context of relationships; it cannot occur in isolation" (p. 133). Contemplating the formulation and engagement of language conducive to healing and reconciliation will oftentimes be a mutual challenge for both the survivor and family members. However, a survivor's engagement in such a dialogue with parents could be the very catalyst needed to help shift both themselves and their families toward a solution-focused healing process.

With a safe therapeutic milieu established, the beginnings of reconnecting family members can begin to take place. Many survivors and their family members alike nurture hopes of reconnection to one another. Herman (1997) emphasizes the role mental health practitioners can play by helping to normalize the survivor and family member responses, feelings, and use of language while always affirming the dignity of the survivor. The willingness for survivors to listen to the story of their parents/caregivers and/or siblings is the other side of the narrative process and an important component of the Empowerment Model. Unfortunately for some survivors of CPSA, because so many years have past since the initial sexual assault, the direct telling to parents may no longer be possible.

Whether parents are deceased, too frail, or unwilling to engage in the exchange, the telling of a survivor's narrative and feeling that one will be heard is needed in the journey of healing for both CPSA survivor and their family members. Identifying creative methods for such an interaction, particularly when a parent may be unavailable due to death or another factor, remains important to all impacted by CPSA.

We have focused on survivor-family reconciliation and healing through the use of the Empowerment Model. However, reconciliation by individuals and families experiencing the impact of CPSA often benefits from a dialogue with the church community's parishioners and church leaders as well. Herman (1997) states,

> Restoration of the breech between the traumatized person and the community depends first upon public acknowledgement of the traumatic event and, second, upon some form of community action. These two responses, recognition and restitution, are necessary to rebuild the survivor's sense of order and justice. (p. 70)

The same is particularly true for survivors and their families of origin, whose primary support system has been the church community. The need for recognition of the wrongs done, understanding, and hope for the future by both the local and larger church community, where so much of the family's identity may have been invested, can be critical for reconciliation and healing and can significantly contribute to the reshaping of family identity and worldview.

CONCLUSION

No two people or their families have identical reactions to traumatic exposure, and this is also true for the trauma of CPSA. In this article, informed by the work of Figley (1989, 1992, 1998) and McCubbin and colleagues (1998), we have considered the experiences of families who have been traumatized by CPSA from the perspective of the survivor. This survivor point of view needs to be expanded to include a direct study of family members, particularly parents and siblings, to further both understanding of the impact of CPSA and development of effective approaches to intervention. We believe the Trauma Transmission and Empowerment models and the FAAR model offer sound theoretical frameworks that could help guide further investigation.

REFERENCES

Antonovsky, A. (1987). *Unraveling the mystery of health.* San Francisco, CA: Jossey-Bass.

Applebaum, D. R., & Burns, G. L. (1991). Unexpected childhood death: Posttraumatic stress disorder in surviving siblings and parents. *Journal of Clinical Child Psychology, 20,* 114–120.

Bera, W. H. (1995). Betrayal: Clergy sexual abuse and male survivors. In J. C. Gonsiorek (Ed.), *Breach of trust: Sexual exploitation by health care professionals and clergy* (pp. 91–111). Thousand Oaks, CA: Sage.

Burkett, E., & Bruni, F. (1993). *A gospel of shame: Children, sexual abuse and the Catholic church.* New York: Viking/Penguin Books.

Cornwell, J., Nurcombe, B., & Stevens, L. (1977). Family response to the loss of a child by sudden infant death syndrome. *Medical Journal of Australia, 1,* 656–658.

Disch, E., & Avery, N. (2001). Sex in the consulting room, the examining room, and sacristy: Survivors of sexual abuse by professionals. *American Journal of Orthopsychiatry, 71*(2), 204–217.

Farrell, D. P., & Taylor, M. (2000). Silenced by God: An examination of unique characteristics within sexual abuse by clergy. *Counselling Psychology Review, 15*(1), 22–31.

Figley, C. R. (1989). *Helping traumatized families.* San Francisco, CA: Jossey-Bass.

Figley, C. R. (1992, June). *Secondary traumatic stress and disorder: Theory, research, and treatment.* Paper presented at the First World Meeting of the International Society for Traumatic Stress Studies, Amsterdam, the Netherlands.

Figley, C. R. (1998). *Burnout in families: The systemic costs of caring.* New York: CRC Press.

Fogler, J. M., Shipherd, J. C., Clarke, S., Jensen, J., & Rowe, E. (2008). The Impact of clergy-perpetrated sexual abuse: The role of gender, development, and posttraumatic stress. *Journal of Child Sexual Abuse, 17*(3–4), 329–358.

Fortune, M. (1989). *Is nothing sacred? When sex invades the pastoral relationship.* San Francisco, CA: Harper and Row.

Gilbert, K. (1998). Understanding the secondary traumatic stress of spouses. In C. R. Figley (Ed.), *Burnout in families: The systemic costs of caring* (pp. 47–74). New York: CRC Press.

Goff, B. S. N., & Schwerdtfeger, K. L. (2004). The systemic impact of traumatized children. In D. R. Catherall (Ed.), *Handbook of stress, trauma, and the family* (pp. 179–202). New York: Brunner-Routledge.

Herman, J. L. (1997). *Trauma and recovery: The aftermath of violence from domestic abuse to political terror.* New York: Basic Books.

Hertz, D.G., & Lerer, B. (1981). The "rape family": Family reactions to the rape victim. *International Journal of Family Psychiatry, 2*(3–4), 301–315.

Isely, P. J. (1996). In their own voices: A qualitative study of men sexually abused as children by Catholic clergy. *Dissertation Abstracts International, 57,* 5328–5329.

Kline, P. M., McMackin, R., & Lezotte, E. (2008). The impact of the clergy abuse scandal on parish communities. *Journal of Child Sexual Abuse, 17*(3–4), 290–300.

Knight, K. (2003). Age of reason. *Catholic encyclopedia* (1907, Vol. 1). New York: Robert Appleton Company.

Manion, I. G., McIntyre, J., Firestone, P., Ligenzinska, M., Ensom, R., & Wells, G. (1996). Secondary traumatization in parents following the disclosure of extrafamilial child sexual abuse: Initial effects. *Child Abuse and Neglect, 20*(11), 1095–1109.

Matsakis, A. (2004). Trauma and its impact on families. In D. R. Catherall (Ed.), *Handbook of stress, trauma, and the family* (pp. 15–31). New York: Brunner-Routledge.

McCubbin, H. I., Thompson, A. I., Thompson, E. A., Elver, K. M., & McCubbin, M. A. (1998). Ethnicity, schema, and coherence: Appraisal processes for families in crisis. In H. I. McCubbin, E. A. Thompson, A. I. Thompson, & J. E. Fromer (Eds.), *Stress, coping, and health in families: Sense of coherence and resiliency* (pp. 41–67). Thousand Oaks, CA: Sage Publications.

Monahon, C. (1993). *Children and trauma: A guide for parents and professionals.* San Francisco, CA: Jossey-Bass.

National Clergy Sex Abuse Report. (2004). *Sexual abuse in social context: Catholic clergy and other professionals.* Special report by the Catholic League for Religious and Civil Rights. Retrieved on March 31, 2007, from http://www.catholicleague.org/research/abuse_in_social_context.htm.

Patterson, J. M., & Garwick, A. W. (1998). Theoretical linkages: Family meanings and sense of coherence. In H. I. McCubbin, E. A. Thompson, A. I. Thompson, & J. E. Fromer (Eds.), *Stress, coping, and health in families: Sense of coherence and resiliency* (pp. 71–89). Thousand Oaks, CA: Sage Publications.

Turnbull, G. J., & McFarlane, A. C. (1996). Acute treatments. In B. van der Kolk, A. McFarlane, & L. Weisaeth (Eds.), *Traumatic stress* (pp. 480–490). New York: Guilford Press.

A Unique Betrayal: Clergy Sexual Abuse in the Context of the Catholic Religious Tradition

Joseph J. Guido

Danny was in eighth grade when it began. Tall for his age and athletic, he was also smart, pious, and dutiful. When Sister told him that Father wanted to see him in the rectory, he left class and walked across the courtyard, ringing the bell and being ushered into a parlor where Father was pacing back and forth. "Thanks for coming, son," Father said as he closed the door to the parlor, "there are several things that I would like to talk with you about." He began talking about high school, the importance of studying hard and of thinking about his future, and the distraction that girls could pose. All the while he paced back and forth while Danny stood still. With each pass in front of Danny, Father would grope his genitals or buttocks and then move on, talking all the while. After a few minutes, Father stopped pacing and unzipped his pants, masturbated in front of Danny, and then dismissed him. Danny returned to class frightened, bewildered, and ashamed.

It happened two more times, once in the church and another time in the sacristy after Mass, and it was always the same: unexpected, accompanied by banal patter, and then nothing—no explanation, no apology, and never a reference to what had taken place. Danny did not tell anyone at the time, shame having gotten the better of him. He was also confused. He knew that what had taken place was wrong and lewd and that he wanted no part of it, but he could not understand why Father, who was otherwise warm and affable and popular with his parishioners, would do such a thing.

In high school and college, Danny drifted away from church and eventually stopped going altogether. He worked hard, received good grades, got a good job when he graduated, and steadily advanced in the company. He also started running. Day after day, he would run mile upon mile and when he could not sleep or when a nightmare would wake him, he would go running in the middle of the night. Running was a comfort, a distraction, and as he knew even then, a metaphor: if he could, he would gladly run away from the memories.

When I first met him, Danny had not seen the inside of a Catholic church in two decades, nor had he spoken with a Catholic priest in that time. We met in a coffee shop, "neutral turf" as Danny called it, and settled into a booth where we talked for the better part of two hours. Danny's therapist thought that telling his story to a priest might be therapeutic for him.

Danny hoped that his story might help others. "Tell them," he insisted, "what he took away from me. Not just my innocence but my faith. I'm like a spiritual orphan, betrayed by what I loved, and I feel lost and alone."

A UNIQUE BETRAYAL: THE DISTINCTIVENESS OF CATHOLIC CULTURE

As Danny's story suggests, the sexual abuse crisis that has roiled the Catholic Church in recent years may be distinguished less by the nature of the crimes, the number of victims, or the complicity of officials than by the particular culture of Catholicism. Often described as a sacramental culture, Catholicism maintains that the created order of people and things manifests an otherwise invisible divine order. For Catholics, this is more than a matter of symbols. The bread and wine used at Mass become the Body and Blood of Christ, and the ordination of a man to the priesthood is no mere deputation or conveyance of office but something that radically changes him. In this sense, the priest-perpetrator is not only a trusted and honored figure but is by virtue of ordination an *alter Christus*, another Christ, and his betrayal of that trust and dishonoring of that role cannot be separated from his sacramental character and meaning. Indeed, precisely because Catholicism suffuses the created order with added meaning, the violation of that order—the violation of an adolescent's body, or of a church or its sacristy—is also a violation of the meaning that it is meant to convey.

But if Catholicism is a sacramental culture, it is also a hierarchical one, and it is the intersection of sacrament and hierarchy that highlights what is distinctively Catholic about the present crisis. Indeed, for many people the greater scandal is that the Church's hierarchy seemingly did too little for too long and thus allowed the abuse to continue. Understandably, many have called for the removal of negligent bishops, greater openness and accountability in church governance and operations, and lay oversight of the church's response to allegations of abuse. Yet for Catholics, such inaction on the part of bishops cannot be considered the ecclesiastical equivalent of corporate malfeasance nor can it be remedied by apology, resignation, and efforts at reform. A bishop's authority derives from that of Christ, and as Christ is the Good Shepherd who would lay down his life for his sheep, so a bishop must act *in personae Christi*—in the person of Christ—and care for his flock even at a price to himself (*Catechism of the Catholic Church*, 1994, nos. 894–896). When he fails to do so, his failure constitutes a betrayal of the sacramental meaning of his authority and leaves his flock, in Danny's words, spiritual orphans.

Thus, in both the immediate experience of the abuse itself and in the extended sense of how the church has responded to it, one cannot understand the effects on survivors and the faithful generally unless one understands the sacramental context in which it took place. Neither can one be of very much assistance if one does not have a measure of cultural competence (American Psychological Association, 2003; Sue & Sue, 2003) specific to Catholicism and sensitive to the interaction between this culture and the lives and experience of individual survivors.

In order to aid this understanding, I will look at Catholic culture from three perspectives. First, I will describe Catholicism in terms of a sacramental worldview that distinguishes it from other denominations and from which quintessentially Catholic rites, rituals, and symbols derive. Second, I will examine the implications of this sacramental worldview for understanding the present crisis. Here I will argue that it is the sacramental understanding of priests and bishops that lends added weight and meaning to the abuse and that may constitute what is unique about the crisis in the Catholic Church. Third, I will suggest ways in which therapists and other caregivers might assist in the repair of sacramental meaning for survivors. Although this may entail a foray into uncharted territory for some professionals, it is not on that account unwarranted and may well be necessary for those survivors whose suffering bears the imprint of a uniquely Catholic culture.

THE SACRAMENTAL WORLDVIEW

The concept of a worldview is intimately associated with that of culture. It encompasses both a fundamental approach to and understanding of the world (Ivey, Ivey, & Simeck-Morgan, 1997; Sue & Sue, 2003) and the corresponding experiences, beliefs, symbols, ethics, rituals, and institutions that constitute a culture (Smart, 2000). It is not just that people in different places and times or from different racial, linguistic, and religious groups act differently, though they do, but that how they think, reason, and are conscious of themselves and others differs. Some would go so far as to argue that "when people live in the world differently, it may be that they live in different worlds" (Shweder, 1991, p. 23).

The Catholic worldview and its corresponding culture can be best understood as sacramental. As a word, *sacramental* shares an etymology with sacrifice and sacrilege, and derives from the Latin for sacred or holy. As a concept, it means that the created order of persons and things can manifest the God who created it. Creation is therefore an act of God's self communication and a means by which to know God (Schulte, 1970). This means that the invisible but necessary and eternal God can be known through and manifest in such contingent and finite realities as bread and wine, and as men who are priests.

Catholics derive this worldview from an understanding of Jesus as God incarnate or "enfleshed." For Catholics and many other Christians, Jesus is fully divine and fully human without compromise of either. It is not that he is God in human form or a human being transformed into God but that he is essentially and necessarily both God and human. This is a statement of faith hard wrung from controversies about his person and nature during the first centuries after his death (Pelikan, 1971), but its import for our purposes is that it establishes a fundamental Catholic typology of the relationship between a sign and what it signifies. Jesus is both the God who is revealed and how that God is revealed most truly, his humanity at one and the same time manifesting his divinity and pointing one to it.

In a similar way, the Catholic Church teaches that its seven sacraments—Baptism, Confirmation, Eucharist, Penance, Marriage, Holy Orders, and the Anointing of the Sick—are the visible signs of invisible grace and the instruments by which that grace is communicated (*Catechism of the Catholic Church*, 1994, no. 774). Thus, even as Jesus is the God he revealed, so the sacraments do what they signify (no. 1127). Confessing one's sins, the laying on of hands, and the exchange of vows are not only signs respectively of forgiveness, priesthood, and marriage but are the very way one is forgiven, becomes a priest, and is joined in marriage. Yet if the sacraments of the Catholic Church effect what they signify, it is not by dint of the faith or worthiness of either the priest or congregation but by virtue of Christ himself (no.1128). It is Christ who is present in the sacraments and he who makes them efficacious even when a priest is sinful and a congregation is only marginally faithful. In this important sense, the sacraments are what they are because they carry on and extend the person and work of Jesus Christ.

This is a bold and singular claim. It is also one that is not limited to the church's seven sacraments. By way of analogy, the church itself can be considered a sacrament since it was founded by Jesus and mediates his person and work (*Catechism of the Catholic Church*, 1994, no. 774; see also Rahner, 1983). There are also ritual actions such as the blessing of medals, the use of holy water, and the exorcising of evil, which the church calls sacramentals. Like the sacraments, sacramentals are signs of grace, but unlike the sacraments, sacramentals are not instruments of grace; that is, they do not effect what they signify (*Catechism of the Catholic Church*, 1994, no. 1167; Lohrer, 1970). Yet despite the nuanced differences between them, the sacraments, the church, and its sacramentals partake of the same worldview in which the things of this earth indicate the things of heaven and, because they do, should be considered holy.

This sacramental worldview has a profound influence on Catholics. It is because of a belief in the capacity of ordinary things and people to manifest the presence and saving activity of God that Catholics genuflect before the tabernacle in a church, containing as it does the wafers of bread that have become the Body and Blood of Christ. It is why Catholics in some cultures and many ethnic groups kiss the hands of a newly ordained priest, believing that he has been transformed by the sacrament of ordination and now bears an indelible mark or character of soul that configures him to Christ as High Priest. It is also ingredient in the church's teaching on the indissolubility of marriage, its preferential option for the poor, and a broad array of artistic and cultural phenomena that partake of what has been called the Catholic imagination (Greeley, 2000).

The sacramental worldview also distinguishes Catholicism from other Christian denominations and from other religions. Although Catholics and protestants share a faith in Jesus as the Son of God, protestants are wont to emphasize God's radical otherness and autonomy, his distance from creation and absence from the world, while Catholics emphasize that God's incarnation in Jesus suggests his nearness to creation and presence to the world (Schloeder, 2003). Similarly, although Jews and Muslims share with Catholics a faith in one God, their consciousness of the holiness and otherness of God prohibits them from fashioning images of the divine. This stands in sharp contrast to Catholics, who use various artistic media to depict God.

The importance and centrality of the sacramental worldview for Catholics is a matter not only of theology but of empirical demonstration. In a recent study of Catholic identity, sociologist Dean Hoge (2002) found that Catholics of every generation rated the sacraments as the most important element in their identification of themselves as Catholic. He asked three generations of Catholics—those born before 1940, those born between 1941–1960, and those born between 1961–1981—to rate more than 20 items associated with being Catholic in terms of their importance to one's identity as a Catholic. In every generational cohort, the sacraments were considered the most important element, and overall 80% of respondents rated them as the most important element. Among those who expressed a higher than average church commitment, the importance of the sacraments was higher still.

These findings are especially notable given how otherwise different these cohorts are. Prior to 1960, Catholic identity in America was often defined in terms of difference, an identity arising from the fact that the Catholic Church was largely a church of immigrants who lived in different neighborhoods and followed different customs from those of their protestant neighbors. One might imagine that the sacraments were just one more instance of difference. Since 1960, however, Catholic identity has evolved along with the improved social and economic status of Catholics and is now best considered in terms of what is distinctive, that is, how Catholics freely choose to define themselves. Yet given the choice, Catholics continue to define themselves in terms of the sacraments. This suggests that the sacramental worldview is deep and persistent among Catholics and is not a consequence of social location but of an enduring self-understanding.

THE IMPLICATIONS OF A SACRAMENTAL WORLDVIEW FOR UNDERSTANDING THE PRESENT CRISIS

The implications of this sacramental worldview for understanding and responding to the sexual abuse crisis in the church should be evident. Given a religious culture in which creation is believed to manifest the divine, the subversion of created reality to evil purposes is a betrayal not only of individuals but of a way of being in the world. This is all the more so when the perpetrator of the abuse is a priest, a man who was himself transformed by the sacrament of Holy Orders into an *alter Christus*, another Christ, and who is entrusted with administering the sacraments to others. In this sense, the sexual abuse of a minor by a priest is a kind of sacrilege that offends against a sacramental worldview and can call it into question.

Many aspects of Danny's experience should be familiar to therapists who have treated survivors of sexual abuse. Fear, confusion and shame, an avoidance of people and places associated with the abuse, difficulty sleeping, disturbing nightmares, and a desire to forget, run away from, and dissociate oneself from the abuse are the common and baleful companions of survival. Yet what is unique about Danny's experience is the effect of the abuse on his faith and his sense of place in the world, leaving him as it did feeling not only betrayed but alone and bereft of the ability to believe. I suggest that this is owed not only to the trauma itself but to the specific and sacramental context in which it occurred. In this way, the sexual abuse of children and adolescents by clergy mirrors what is true of trauma generally: namely, that while its general effects are continuous across persons and circumstances, its specific effects reflect the culture and meaning that attends on it.

Judith Herman (1981, 1992) and Jonathan Shay (1994) illustrate this point in their respective treatments of domestic and combat trauma. Herman argues that domestic violence and war affect people in similar ways but that, historically, the public response to allegations of incest and rape has been skeptical, often dismissive of victims, and forgetful of the truths that they tell. As a result, victims of incest and rape are symptomatic in specific and commensurate ways. They are prone to neglect their own safety, are likely to be traumatized repeatedly, often second guess themselves, and doubt that they are worthy of anything good, noble, and tender. Not having been taken seriously, they often find it difficult to take themselves seriously.

On the other hand, Shay (1994) details how men caught in the very public throes of war are commonly traumatized by their intimate losses: the death of a friend or betrayal by officers who, like incestuous fathers, fail to protect those entrusted to their care and rather lend them to ignoble purposes. Here it is the implicit bonds between men and the dependency and responsibility that they inspire that serve as the hidden context for combat. Not uncommonly, therefore, traumatized veterans withdraw from normal social engagement, shoulder onerous guilt for having survived when others did not and only at the price of all that is good and decent, and are inclined to displace their anguish and rage onto others. Indeed, it is hard to reestablish connections with others when the very possibility of connection has been violently betrayed.

When the church describes a priest or bishop as an *alter Christus* who should act *in personae Christi*, it locates sexual abuse by priests in a very specific and powerful context of meaning. Indeed, from its first centuries until now the Catholic Church has understood that the sacrament of Holy Orders changes a man fundamentally and permanently and leaves him uniquely able to act in the name and in the person of Christ (Hussey,1991; Osborne, 1988). Thus, the *Catechism of the Catholic Church* (1994) emphasizes the conveyance of a sacred character and power to the priest through ordination (no. 1538), its essential difference from that conveyed by other sacraments (no. 1547), its permanence (no. 1583), and, as a result, the priest's special conformity to Christ (no. 1563).

To be sure, this understanding of priesthood represents centuries of development during which the emphasis differed according to the times. The Council of Trent (1545–1563), occurring as it did during the Reformation, was keen to distinguish Catholic and protestant theological positions and so emphasized the cultic aspects of priesthood to the exclusion of others (Osborne, 1988). Thus, the priest was different and special, defined by his sacramental activity and his role in the sacrifice of the Mass, and his distinction was signified by the manner of his dress, his specialized education, and his place of residence. This view held sway until the Second Vatican Council (1962–1965). Vatican II, as it is commonly known, rejoined the cultic aspects of priesthood—the priest's role in worship and the sacraments—to those aspects that Trent had largely neglected. Thus a priest is to be understood not only in terms of his role at Mass but also in terms of his pastoral care of others (Power, 1999), his collaboration with the bishops and other priests in building up the unity of the Church (Kasper, 1969), and in terms of his witness to and proclamation of the Gospel (John Paul II, 1992).

Yet the consistent teaching that a priest is different precisely in the sense of being specially conformed to Christ suggests an important way in which abuse by priests is different from that perpetrated by others. A priest's status and authority derive not from his gender or his status as husband or father, nor from brute strength or size nor from his attainment of rank, but from Christ. In this way, the effects of clerical abuse take on a specifically religious and existential cast that helps to explain Danny's experience. Danny was left without faith, alone and spiritually orphaned in part because his abuse cannot be understood without reference to the sacramental context in which Father was a man of God uniquely enabled to represent Christ and to make him present. That such a man would abuse him cannot but give rise to questions about the nature and reality of God, the veracity of his love, care, and protection, and Danny's place in the economy of salvation. It also evokes the paradox at the heart of the sacramental worldview.

To assert that finite, created reality can manifest the divine and infinite is to contradict appearances, and the present crisis in the Catholic Church has made plain the inadequacy of ordinary men to do so. Yet what appears to be a contradiction should be understood in light of the church's fundamental realism. The *Catechism of the Catholic Church* (1994, no. 1148) quotes both the Council of Trent and St. Thomas Aquinas (1964) to the effect that the sacraments act *ex opere operato*, that is, by virtue of Christ's action and not the worthiness of the priest or recipient. It is not that the sacraments are magical or that priests should not try to live up to the holiness of Christ to whom they have been configured by ordination; rather it is only Christ who can do what needs to be done, be it to forgive sins, consecrate bread and wine as his Body and Blood, or take an ordinary man and make him a priest.

That is why the Catholic Church teaches that the change effected by ordination is ontological rather than moral. A priest is an *alter Christus* because Christ has configured his being to his own, but whether he is morally Christ-like is quite a different thing and not, technically speaking, necessary for Christ to use him sacramentally. At heart, this is a statement about the fidelity of Christ despite the infidelity of his priests and can perhaps be best appreciated negatively. If Christ's sacramental presence— in Mass, in Confession—depended on the goodness and holiness of the priest, then it could well be a rare thing, but if it depends on the holiness and goodness of Christ then it can be true despite the failings of the priest.

In this way, priest perpetrators have indeed grossly violated their sacramental character and the intention of Christ in choosing them as priests, and may have severely compromised people's ability to experience Christ's sacramental presence. But they have not thereby obviated that sacramental presence of Christ nor have they, in the most radical sense, contradicted the sacramental worldview. Indeed, properly understood, this worldview requires that creation be inadequate to its task even when creation is at its best for we hold this treasure in earthen vessels (1 Corinthians 4:6–8). This is not to excuse priest perpetrators nor their negligent bishops—far from it. But it is to suggest that the Church's boldness in asserting the sacramental worldview is matched by its realism.

One measure of this realism can be found in a study of how Catholics reacted to an earlier wave of sexual abuse by priests (Rossetti, 1994). Among Catholics who had not personally experienced abuse by a priest, exposure varied from minimal (reading about it or hearing news accounts) to rather more intimate acquaintance, as when one's parish or family were affected. Not surprisingly, the more intimate their exposure the more likely it was that Catholics would lose trust in the priesthood and the Catholic Church (see Kline, McMackin, & Lezotte, 2008). This was not true of their trust in God, however, which remained unchanged across levels of exposure. It is as if the sacramental worldview that allows created and finite reality to manifest the divine also allows for the fact that the failings of the former need not compromise the integrity of the latter.

ASSISTING IN THE REPAIR OF SACRAMENTAL MEANING

Danny needed good and competent clinical care, which he was fortunate to receive. It helped to attenuate the nightmares, the sudden flares of fear and anger, and the persistent sense that he was somehow though inexplicably to blame for what had happened. He had a good marriage and was a good father, and all things considered had a good life. Yet he remained a spiritual orphan. For people like Danny, healing cannot be limited to the remediation of dysfunction and the alleviation of symptoms but must attend to the religious challenges implied by the abuse. Paramount among these is the challenge to a sacramental worldview and its attendant meaning.

In recent years, there has been a spate of interest in religion and mental health (Koenig, 1998; Miller, 1999; Richards & Bergin, 1997, 2000; Shafranske, 1996), and though mental health professionals tend to be less religious than the clients they serve, there has been greater openness to attending to clients' spiritual needs as part of a comprehensive treatment plan (see Pargament, Murray-Swank, & Mahoney, 2008). Nevertheless, clinicians appear to be rather more at ease addressing spirituality broadly considered than religion per se, and there is a paucity of studies about the collaboration between mental health professionals and clergy (McMinn & Chaddock, 2003; Weaver, Flannelly, Flannelly, & Oppenheimer, 2003). Indeed, there are far more studies addressing how to facilitate clergy referrals to clinicians than how clinicians might refer to clergy.

In working with survivors of clergy abuse, it is important therefore for clinicians to be acquainted with the particular sacramental culture of Catholicism, the basic theology noted, and to be able to refer survivors to competent and sensitive representatives of the Catholic Church if and when they request it. Sometimes it is sufficient to be acquainted with a diocese's office of pastoral outreach to survivors or, alternately, its advisory board for the protection of children and youth. In the absence of personal familiarity with these offices and individuals, information can be obtained by visiting the official Web site of the United States Conference of Catholic Bishops (www.usccb.org) and then linking to the appropriate diocesan webpage.

At other times, it is important to be able to refer survivors to individuals who can help them address directly the religious and spiritual implications of their experience. This can be a difficult task. Distinguishing between subjective experience of the sacred and its objective manifestation is never easy and is made all the more difficult when the two are conflated in the person of the priest-perpetrator. Yet this is the task of the *cura animarum* or care of souls. This refers to the ancient tradition of the Catholic Church in which a confessor or spiritual director provides moral and spiritual guidance and whose unique charge is to attend to one's experience of and relationship with God (Barry & Connolly, 1983). Although confessors are priests, spiritual directors may be priests, religious or lay people, male or female, and in addition to appropriate education and training should manifest a sense of special calling and talent for this work.

It is also important to consider that the repair of sacramental meaning may take different forms at different times with different people. In his landmark study of religious forms of coping, Kenneth Pargament (1997) distinguished successful forms of coping from those that are unsuccessful. Religious ritual, prayer, and switching from one church or denomination to another may or may not help, and persistently angry, blaming, and negative framing of God's role in the adversity surely does not. Nor is it a matter that religious forms of coping are merely variants on social support and cognitive reframing. Although successful religious coping entails the use of social supports and cognitive reframing, it adds a dimension to coping that is unique and irreducible and one that cannot be supplied by other resources. What successful religious coping does is help individuals find meaning and significance in the midst of adversity, and this with reference to the sacred. Ordinarily and nearly always at first, people attempt to find meaning and significance by returning to what they have known and what has worked for them in the past. Pargament calls this the conservation of significance and maintains that often it works quite well. There are experiences of adversity, however, that overwhelm our ability to conserve meaning and significance, and that rather call for its transformation. Calamities, natural disasters, and trauma often exceed our customary ways of making sense of the world, and if our only recourse is what we have known and it fails us, then our grasp on God can seem tenuous indeed.

The transformation of meaning and significance is not easy, requires the ability to weather transition and uncertainty, and entails a transformation of the self en route. Indeed, one must undergo a spiritual conversion—something quite different than a switch in denomination—in which one finds God anew, at a more profound and personal level, and with a keen appreciation for the heretofore unacknowledged limitations of the self and the unlikely prospect of forgiving the unforgivable. It would not be surprising to find that for some survivors of sexual abuse by priests this is precisely the challenge they confront. It is not only that their sense of the sacred may have failed them at their time of greatest need but that the sacred itself has seemingly been the agent of their betrayal and harm. It is the sacred therefore that must be found anew if it is to be preserved. And within the ambit of Catholic culture, it is the sacramental that is the needed medium for that rediscovery.

Some survivors may conclude that the sacred is not worth rediscovering. Others will find it in new venues and apart from the Catholic Church. But some will seek it where it was betrayed. If they are to find it, they must find us willing companions for the journey, tolerant both of their need to find what has been lost and of their wariness to do so. We must also be tolerant of the real limitations of the created order to fulfill what it is charged to do, namely, to manifest and point the way to the divine. In doing so, we join survivors in the journey to find the holy in the profane, the infinite in the irrefutably limited, and God in what is all too human. As Dante knew well, the passage through hell to heaven is not meant to be undertaken alone but only in the company of those gentle guides who are willing to make the journey with us.

CONCLUSION

Danny died in the fall of 2004. I read his obituary in the newspaper. It described his work, his family, and his interests, and the calling hours for his wake. It also noted that his funeral service would be conducted at a local church, although not a Catholic one. He was young, just shy of 40, and though I had heard that he had cancer I could not help but wonder what toll the abuse had taken on his health. But what moved me most was the fact that he had found his way back to church. I do not know whether he had been attending regularly or what it meant about his faith, only that it was not the "neutral turf" we had met on and that he would not be alone. Spiritual orphan though he was, he would not pass from this world alone. Family and friends and congregants would gather around him, sing and pray and bless him, and see him safely to his resting place. In good Catholic fashion, I said a prayer for him and for all of the dead, believing as I do that we are all of us, living and deceased, part of a single communion that is at one and the same time blessed and broken, holy and sinful, a sacrament as it were of the triumph of grace over all.

REFERENCES

American Psychological Association. (2003). *Ethical principles of psychologists and code of conduct.* Washington, DC: Author.

Barry, W. & Connolly, W. (1983). *The practice of spiritual direction.* New York: Seabury.

Catechism of the Catholic Church. (1994). Mahwah, NJ: Paulist Press.

Greeley, A. (2000). *The Catholic imagination.* Berkeley, CA: University of California Press.

Herman, J. (1981). *Father-daughter incest.* Cambridge, MA: Harvard University Press.

Herman, J. (1992). *Trauma and recovery.* Cambridge, MA: Harvard University Press.

Hoge, D. (2002). Core and periphery in American Catholic identity. *Journal of Contemporary Religion, 17*(3), 293–302.

Hussey, M. (1991). The priesthood after the council: Theological reflections. In K. Smith (Ed.), *Priesthood in the modern world* (pp. 19–28). Franklin, WI: Sheed & Ward.

Ivey, A., Ivey, M., & Simek-Morgan, L. (1997). *Counseling and psychotherapy: A multicultural perspective* (4th ed.). Boston: Allyn & Bacon.

John Paul II. (1992). *Pastoro Dabo Vobis.* Retrieved January 2, 2004, from http://www. vatican.va/holy_father/john_paul_ii.

Kasper, W. (1969). A new dogmatic outlook on priestly ministry. In K. Rahner (Ed.), *The identity of the priest* (pp. 20–33). New York: Paulist Press.

Kline, P. M., McMackin, R., & Lezotte, E. (2008). The impact of the clergy abuse scandal on parish communities. *Journal of Child Sexual Abuse, 17*(3–4), 290–300.

Koenig, H. (Ed.). (1998). *Handbook of religion and mental health.* New York: Academic Press.

Lohrer, M. (1970). Sacramentals. In K. Rahner (Ed.), *Sacramentum Mundi* (Vol. 5, pp. 375–378). New York: Herder & Herder.

McMinn, M., & Chaddock. T. (2003). Psychologists collaboration with clergy. *Professional Psychology: Research & Practice, 29*(6), 564–578.

Miller, W. (Ed.) (1999). *Integrating spirituality into treatment.* Washington, DC: American Psychological Association.

Osborne, K. (1988). *A history of the ordained ministry in the Roman Catholic church.* New York: Paulist Press.

Pargament, K. (1997). *The psychology of religion and coping.* New York: Guilford Press.

Pargament, K., Murray-Swank, N., & Mahoney, A. (2008). Problem and solution: The spiritual dimension of clergy sexual abuse and its impact on survivors. *Journal of Child Sexual Abuse, 17*(3–4), 397–420.

Pelikan, J. (1971). *The emergence of the Catholic tradition (100–600).* Chicago: University of Chicago Press.

Power, D. (1999). Evolution of the priesthood: Adapting to pastoral needs. In K. Smith (Ed.), *Priesthood in the modern world* (pp. 29–38). Franklin, WI: Sheed & Ward.

Rahner, K. (1983). *Foundations of Christian faith.* William Dych (Trans.). New York: Crossroad/Herder & Herder.

Richards, S., & Bergin, A. (Eds.) (1997). *A spiritual strategy for counseling and psychotherapy.* Washington, DC: American Psychological Association.

Richards, S., & Bergin, A. (Eds.) (2000). *Handbook of psychotherapy and religious diversity.* Washington, DC: American Psychological Association.

Rossetti, S. (1994). The effects of priest perpetration of child sexual abuse on the trust of Catholics in priesthood, Church and God. *Dissertation Abstracts International, 55*(06), 2389.

Schloeder, S. (2003). Sacred architecture and the Christian imagination. In K. Whitehead (Ed.), *The Catholic imagination* (pp.74–96). South Bend, IN: St. Augustine's Press.

Schulte, R. (1970). Sacraments. In K. Rahner (Ed.), *Sacramentum Mundi* (Vol. 5, pp. 378–384). New York: Herder & Herder.

Shafranske, E. (Ed.) (1996). *Religion and the clinical practice of psychology.* Washington, DC: American Psychological Association.

Shay, J. (1994). *Achilles in Vietnam.* New York: Atheneum.

Shweder, R. (1991). *Thinking through cultures: Expeditions in cultural psychology.* Cambridge, MA: Harvard University Press.

Smart, N. (2000). *Worldviews: Crosscultural explorations of human beliefs.* Upper Saddle River, NJ: Prentice Hall.

St. Thomas Aquinas. (1964). *Summa theologiae.* (T. Gilby, Ed. and Trans.). New York and Oxford: McGraw-Hill/Blackfriars.

Sue, D. W., & Sue, D. (2003). *Counseling the culturally diverse: Theory and practice.* New York: John Wiley & Sons.

Weaver, A., Flannelly, K., Flannelly, L., & Oppenheimer, J. (2003). Collaboration between clergy and mental health professionals: A review of professional health care journals from 1980 through 1999. *Counseling & Values, 47*(3), 162–172.

A Single-Case Study of Rabbinic Sexual Abuse in the Orthodox Jewish Community

Amy Neustein
Michael Lesher

Judaism is a monotheistic but not a monolithic faith. There are three major religious branches within Judaism: Orthodox, Conservative, and Reform. These are roughly differentiated by descending degrees of adherence to traditional Jewish law. This paper examines an individual case of reported child sexual abuse (CSA) where the alleged perpetrator was an Orthodox rabbi from a strict adherence community. Such communities are sometimes referred to as "ultra-Orthodox," "hareidi," or "Hasidic." While this case highlights some of the conflicts inherent when traditional Jewish systems of justice interact with secular systems of justice, it is not meant to be an attack on such traditional systems of justice. The authors are Orthodox Jews who present this material to foster greater understanding of the broad themes they believe this case represents.

THE RABBINIC COURT PROCEDURE

Several years ago, a prominent Orthodox Jewish psychologist expressed his concern over the handling of CSA cases in his religious community in an open letter to a major Jewish newspaper:

> [I]f the police do get involved [in a CSA case], a massive cover-up and pressure campaign usually ensures that the case will either not get to trial or if it does, will be dropped because potential witnesses are pressured (code for threatened) to refuse to testify or outright lie. (Glick, 2000, pp. 87–88)

The "pressure campaign" this psychologist described is enhanced by a social institution largely peculiar to Orthodox Jewish communities: the rabbinic court, or *beth din*. Jewish tradition traces these courts all the way back to Moses. Historically, rabbinic courts have "exerted full and unchallenged authority" over Jewish communal life in many areas, "as in trade, real estate dealings, torts and damages, marriage and divorce," as far back as third century Babylonia (Neusner, 1970, p. 447). To this day, traditionally observant Jews regard it as a sin, except under clearly defined circumstances, to take their disputes to a non-Jewish court in preference to a *beth din*. As a result, Orthodox Jews often present conflicts involving business, community politics, neighborhood quarrels, or marital disharmony to a rabbinic court for resolution (see *Shulhan Arukh, Hoshen ha-Mishpat* 26:1 *et seq*).

Given the religious imperative behind them, rabbinic courts have great prestige in Orthodox Jewish communities, and this in turn can blind these communities to the severe limitations under which such courts necessarily labor when dealing with criminal or antisocial conduct. In fact, rabbinic courts are largely impotent to control actions such as CSA since they are unable to arrest suspects, compel the production of information or evidence, detain a suspect pending the outcome of a trial, or punish an offender in the event he or she is found guilty. Nevertheless, for reasons to be examined in more detail, Orthodox Jews often take concerns about possible CSA to a rabbinic court for "resolution" before engaging secular authorities. This leads to a paradox: rabbinic courts, which can do little or nothing to deal with an offender who is "convicted," can still wield great influence if their verdict favors the accused, as victims and potential witnesses alike may be threatened with ostracism or worse on religious grounds if they subsequently take their grievances to the police or testify in a criminal trial.

This effectively results in a lopsided balance of power between accuser and accused in rabbinic courts where the accuser has little or nothing to gain no matter what happens, while the accused stands to gain a great deal from a favorable outcome. Frequently, Orthodox rabbis being prosecuted for CSA by secular authorities have often simultaneously engaged rabbinic courts to investigate the same charges. In some of these cases, on reaching a verdict of "not guilty" the rabbis who make up the *beth din* have changed their roles from judges to advocates for the accused, approaching secular authorities to urge the dismissal of a criminal charge, which can result in exactly the "cover-up" Dr. Glick described in the letter quoted previously.

This article explores the way a rabbinic court intervened in a Brooklyn case involving serious charges of child abuse embodied in a 96-count complaint. After the members of the rabbinic court conducted their own "trial" and pressured secular authorities to accept their verdict of "not guilty," the criminal complaint was abruptly withdrawn while the case was still being presented to a grand jury. The details of what happened in this case offer significant insights into both the *beth din* legal process as administered by the Orthodox rabbinate and the mechanics by which its attitudes toward CSA, non-Jews, secular adjudication, and concern over public scandal can cloud the workings of the criminal justice system.

"INFORMING": A HISTORICAL AND SOCIOLOGICAL PROBLEM FOR JEWISH COMMUNITIES

While the case to be discussed in this paper was being processed, a full-page notice was published in a community Yiddish newspaper bearing a "severe prohibition and serious warning" against making police reports even against a suspected child abuser. This notice, written in the formal Hebrew of the traditional religious texts, was supported by the names of 50 prominent rabbis as cosignatories. It stated:

> A Jewish man or woman who informs [to non-Jewish authorities], saying, "I shall go and inform upon another Jew," with respect to either his property or person, and [such person] was warned not to inform and he demurs and insists, "I shall inform!"—regarding him, it is a *mitzvah* [positive commandment] to kill him and whoever has the first opportunity to kill him is entitled to do so, as in the law of the "pursuer" [the law that permits killing someone who is attempting to kill someone else]. ("Notice," 2000, p. 8)

This passage, in rough outline, is based on a seminal 16th century authority for practical Jewish law, *Shulhan Arukh, Hoshen ha-Mishpat* 388:9. The roots of the law extend to the Talmudic legislation of the early Middle Ages (e.g., Babylonian Talmud *Baba Kamma* 116b–117a and *Gittin* 7a). However, neither the Talmud nor the traditional law codes actually define a police report regarding a suspected criminal as "informing" within the meaning of the prohibition.

The license to kill, in particular, will startle many outsiders to the Jewish community, even in those cases religious law does define as "informing." It is best understood as a reflection of the bitter experience of Jews at the hands of many non-Jewish governments, which has led to extreme hostility toward "informers" and an ingrained cultural habit of avoiding dealing with secular government wherever possible. A natural concomitant to this attitude is the harsh punishment threatened to those who violate the prohibition. Thus, the concept of *m'sirah* and its accompanying death penalty have been invoked, even in modern times, to protect Jews from malicious talebearing to hostile authorities. For instance, it is reported that a Jew who was suspected of passing information to the Soviet NKVD (People's Commissariat of Internal Affairs) was threatened with death in order to protect members of his community from potentially deadly military service during World War II (*The Rebbes*, 1993).

The horror traditional Jews have come to feel toward *m'sirah*, after centuries of grim experience, has increasingly come to dictate policies among Orthodox Jews regarding reporting a rabbi suspected of CSA. Neither the phenomenon of sex abuse cover-ups in general in religious Jewish communities nor the details of the case we present can be understood apart from this ingrained traditional resistance to the engagement of secular authorities.

The traditional Jewish mistrust for secular authorities is by no means restricted to sex abuse investigations. In February 1993 and reported in the *New York Times* in 1994, the Department of Education investigated widespread Pell grant fraud in the New York area, issuing subpoenas to schools and individuals who were suspected of running sham postsecondary school programs with federal money (Winerip, 1994). For months, full-page ads ran in prominent Jewish newspapers, signed by eminent rabbis, urging special "sensitivity" on the part of government officials when serving subpoenas on Orthodox Jews. The rabbis, who were able to secure the support of several United States senators from the region, wanted the Jewish schools to receive advance notice before federal agents arrived with subpoenas to seize their records. They argued that an unannounced visit would be especially traumatic for Jews given their recent history in Eastern Europe, where hostile non-Jewish government authorities would conduct "ambush" searches of their homes for incriminating evidence.

Not every Orthodox rabbi supports the cultural prejudice that makes traditional Jews reluctant to turn to government authorities, particularly when a crime such as CSA is suspected. Rabbi Mark Dratch, a leading authority on Jewish clerical abuse, has publicly rejected the invocation of *m'sirah* to shield a rabbi accused of abuse from being reported to secular authorities. Speaking at a "roundtable" of the Rabbinic Council of America, Rabbi Dratch (1992) argued that *m'sirah* is misapplied in cases of CSA, in which the overriding obligation of *pikuah nefesh* (saving a life or, as here, a functioning soul) should take precedence over any concern about reporting a Jew to secular authorities.

However, the issue is not simply one of religious law. Rabbi Dratch himself, in discussing the misapplication of *m'sirah*, has pointed to factors that still motivate members of Orthodox communities to protect pedophiles and sexual offenders from criminal investigation and prosecution. For example, Rabbi Dratch notes the fear among his coreligionists that a suspected rabbi, if jailed, may be attacked in prison. Another commonly expressed fear is that the convicted rabbi's family name will be so badly tarnished that his children and relatives will have difficulty finding suitable marriage partners.

These concerns touch on yet another motive traditional Jewish communities have for avoiding police reports. This is the preoccupation of such communities with the fear of scandal. Orthodox Jewish communities are extremely self-conscious about public image—partly because of religious doctrine that makes them responsible, on the basis of their behavior, for the reputation of the God they serve (see *Mishnah, Aboth* 4:5), and partly because of historically grounded fears that scandal can reinforce anti-Semitism and give enemies of the Jews an excuse to attack. The publicity attracted by a charge of CSA against a rabbi is therefore considered as bad as the act itself. As a result, it is not unusual for members of Orthodox communities to "publicly defend [a religious Jew] just to keep him out of the criminal justice system," as one insider explained to the authors (personal communication, July 10, 2000). This can have profound consequences for victims of CSA. For example, in 1990, prominent rabbis allegedly threw their weight behind a Hasidic operator of a Brooklyn day care center after he was accused by parents of having molested children in his care. A friend of one of those parents complained to *The Jewish Week* that "they [the rabbis] have an 'in' with the District Attorney's office and hold weight as to whether a case is pressed or not. They want this one shoved under the carpet . . . so it is going to be hushed up" (Ain, 1990, p. 7). In the end, that is exactly what happened.

In spite of authoritative rulings such as those of Rabbi Dratch, the strong sociological factors described previously cause most Orthodox Jews to shield abusers from authorities. Some cases described to the authors involve public attacks or the threat of such attacks on the character or credibility of the accuser in order to suppress an accusation. In other cases, someone credibly accused of CSA is quietly expelled from his or her local community. Neither course protects prospective victims or vindicates children who have already been abused. Even if an accused predator is banished from one community, he or she can almost always find another one, since the predator escapes official law enforcement investigation and is never prosecuted, let alone punished, for his or her actions.

The case examined in this article involves a paradoxical twist on this theme. In this case, because the family of the alleged victim *did* turn to the police, the members of a rabbinic court approached the secular prosecutors as well, not to cooperate with the prosecution but in order to cut it short. They succeeded. Thus, hostility to secular authorities led rabbis from the Orthodox Jewish community, in the end, to manipulate those authorities with the result that a credibly accused child abuser went free.

The discussion of this case, therefore, illuminates sociological patterns that reach beyond the details of a particular incident. This case forces us to consider the effects of religious culture, history, mistrust of outsiders, and fear of scandal on a community that has risen to political prominence in several urban areas in the United States. As this example shows, the social mores at work in this community can cause rabbis and Jewish community members to obstruct the prosecution of sex crimes committed by rabbis, whether in temples, synagogues, day schools, or yeshivas.[1]

CASE MATERIAL

Case Selection Criteria

The authors chose this particular case for in-depth research and reporting for three reasons. First, the case involved important figures and political groups. The accused and accuser belonged to one of the world's largest Hasidic sects, which in New York has become a powerful voting bloc. The rabbi accused of abuse enlisted the services of a nationally recognized trial attorney. The case was initially given high-profile treatment by the Brooklyn district attorney (DA), and it received prompt television coverage. And, as we will show, it generated a very strong reaction within the Orthodox Jewish community. Second, this case brought together rabbis from an unusually broad array of Orthodox communities to serve as arbiters. Consequently, it illustrates that the forces that derailed this particular CSA prosecution belong not just to one ultra-Orthodox sect, but to many segments of this population. Third, the details and outcome of the case continue to resonate in the collective memory of the more progressive mental health professionals within the Orthodox Jewish community, whether or not these professionals were personally connected with it.

Interview Procedures

While investigating this case history as journalists, the authors employed appropriate journalistic standards, which are congruent with human subject research standards in the social sciences. The authors took care to protect the rights, welfare, and integrity of their human subjects. The 13-month study of the facts began with interviews of a doctor and a speech therapist involved in the case from whom the authors sought guidance as to how best to approach the victim's family. Only after the professionals contacted the family and the family granted permission to proceed did the authors contact family members. Moreover, before interviewing the victim's family members, the authors conferred with a mental health professional about the questions to be posed to the subjects.

The authors have not used the actual name of the victim or of his family members and have provided anonymity to other sources who asked that their names be withheld. In keeping with the standards used by social researchers, the authors also excluded details about the alleged offender's political affiliations, family/political connections, personal history, etc.

During the course of the case study, the authors conducted numerous interviews, many of them long, often at late hours of the night, to accommodate the prayer and teaching schedules of the rabbis who agreed to be interviewed. The authors followed a careful procedure for interviewing subjects. Before each interview, they reviewed with one another a list of prepared questions; following each interview, they compared notes via detailed e-mail and phone discussions. Some interviews were joint face-to-face meetings. For some subjects (victim's family members, community members, the alleged offender's wife, rabbinic supporters), interviews by a single author were often deemed preferable, particularly where two interviewers could have induced unnecessary stress in the subject. To reduce contamination of data, the authors shared and reviewed the transcripts of each interview with one another. This procedure helped the authors to maintain a scientific approach to an emotionally charged project.

The authors were at pains to make sure that this case did not present an anomaly, such as a victim with a mental disorder or an offender who had a historical or consanguineous relationship with the family of the victim so as to ensure that the research findings would not be skewed by such factors. In addition, to ensure that the findings were corroborated, notwithstanding the qualitative approach employed, the authors interviewed many sources besides the ones cited in the article. For example, the authors interviewed rabbis who presided over other rabbinic panels, Orthodox Jewish therapists and medical doctors, Orthodox community members and leaders, religious schoolteachers, and others. However, the authors understand the limitations of such single subject qualitative methods and do not claim that this case is necessarily representative of all cases of clergy abuse within the Jewish community.

Case History

In January 2000, Rabbi Solomon Hafner, a member of the Bobov Hasidic sect in Brooklyn, New York, was arrested and charged with first and second degree child abuse for allegedly twisting and tugging a young boy's genitals over eighteen months of religious tutoring.

Barely two months after Rabbi Hafner's arrest, the office of Brooklyn DA Charles "Joe" Hynes, after a visit from a member of an influential panel of ultra-Orthodox rabbis, abruptly announced that "there is no evidence to support the charges" (Kings County District Attorney's Office, 2000). The charges against Rabbi Hafner were then dropped and the grand jury that had been hearing testimony in the case disbanded.

Members of Brooklyn's ultra-Orthodox community have expressed little doubt about who got the DA to dismiss the Hafner case. "We educated the DA on how to properly conduct a sex abuse trial," stated Rabbi Chaim Rottenberg, one of the rabbinic judges whose court cleared Hafner, to the authors. "If we didn't convince the DA," Rabbi Rottenberg asked *The Jewish Voice and Opinion* rhetorically, "then why did Hynes drop the case so suddenly?" (Rosenbluth, 2006, p. 16).

"This [the Bobov Hasidim and their supporters] is a very powerful, political community," said Katherine Grimm, the pediatrician and child abuse expert who examined the alleged victim and then turned the case over to the police. "The community [rank and file] was told not to talk to the police . . . [And] there were definitely things said about [the boy and his family] that weren't true." In the end, said Grimm, "justice was obstructed."[2]

The history of the charges against Hafner certainly appears to describe a legitimate case. In 1997, "David Abraham" (not his real name) was nine years old. Because of his serious hearing deficiency, he required special tutoring in order to be "mainstreamed" into the Bobov yeshiva, or religious school, where he was a student. Rabbi Solomon Hafner seemed a natural choice for the job. According to his wife, the 38-year-old Hafner, with nine children of his own, had tutored "hundreds" of other children in the Bobov community over 18 years, and he was well known to the Abraham family. "I never fought with [the Abrahams]," remembered Chaya Hafner, Rabbi Hafner's wife, who says she was shocked when her husband was charged with abuse. "[We were] friendly, good friends, knew each other for years."

The tutoring took place from eight to nine on weekday mornings in a converted house known as the Voydislaver Synagogue. This location was chosen, according to Mrs. Hafner, because it was "secluded" and thus best suited to the boy's special needs. But during a year and a half of intensive tutoring from Hafner, the boy's performance, to his parents' surprise, seemed rather to stagnate than to improve. "He was daydreaming, distracted," says his speech pathologist, Adele Markwitz. This was particularly puzzling to the family since the boy, notwithstanding his hearing problem, was described by Markwitz as "very intelligent and hardwork-ing." In late 1998, "worried about his behavior and performance," accord-ing to Dr. Grimm, the parents fired Rabbi Hafner as their son's tutor. But no one yet suspected abuse.

Months later, the boy began to disclose bizarre details of his 18 months with Rabbi Hafner. "They were sadistic things," Grimm told the authors, audibly balancing outrage and professional detachment. "Pulling of his genitals . . . hitting the ear with the hearing aid." The child also said he was threatened with worse than this if he told anyone about the abuse.

Grimm confirmed that Mrs. Abraham, like other Hasidim, was so reluctant to allow charges like these into general view that she spent over eight months seeking a solution "within the community." "The mother's concern [was] for other children who may be at risk," she says. "She felt it was her ethical duty."

Finding her fellow Hasidim uninterested in her concerns, Mrs. Abraham finally decided that intervention from "outside" was necessary. Armed with the support of two Orthodox Jewish therapists, Meir Wikler and Moshe Wangrofsky, both of whom reportedly believed the boy was tell-ing the truth, Mrs. Abraham had her son examined by Dr. Grimm, who worked with the Manhattan Children's Advocacy Center, and who, as an assistant professor at Mount Sinai Medical Center, not only chaired a child abuse clinical evaluation program but taught other doctors about child abuse prevention and detection. Grimm was impressed: "The boy's story was consistent to everyone he spoke to and in all the details."

Detective Brenda Vincent Springer of the New York Police Depart-ment's (NYPD) Special Victims Squad, described by Dr. Grimm as an experienced professional with specific experience in the Hasidic Jewish community, interviewed the child after Grimm made an official report of suspected abuse. "She [Springer] found the [boy's] story to be very credi-ble," said Grimm. "She was so encouraging, and she was so helpful," said Mrs. Abraham of Detective Springer. "My son felt so secure with her, like she really understood him, and he wasn't scared to tell her what actually happened, like he told her things that he hadn't even told us happened." (Springer was barred by NYPD rules from commenting to the authors.)

After Rabbi Hafner's arrest on January 13, however, the reaction in Bobov was swift and angry. Kevin Davitt, the Brooklyn DA's Director of Public Information, acknowledged that some members of the Bobov community complained to his office that the DA was on a "witch hunt" against Hasidim. Henna White, the DA's official liaison to Orthodox Jews, went farther than that: she said that after Rabbi Hafner was formally charged, she heard from "sources" that even Dovid Cohen, a prominent Brooklyn rabbi who had approved the Abrahams' resort to secular author-ities, had been "threatened."

Intervention of a Beth Din

The key to what happened in the Hafner case is found in understanding the *beth din*, which was assembled in February 2000 in response to Bobov community pressure to make its own "inside" investigation of the charges against Rabbi Hafner. The rabbinic court was composed of five rabbis drawn from ultra-Orthodox communities all over New York City and its surrounding territory. At its head was Manhattan's Rabbi Dovid Feinstein, the son of one of America's most famous Orthodox rabbis, the late Moshe Feinstein. From the very beginning, at least one member of the court, Rabbi Chaim Rottenberg, chief rabbi of a Hasidic enclave in Monsey, a heavily ultra-Orthodox community 35 miles from Manhattan, clearly saw the rabbinic panel as a way to try to influence the official legal proceed-ings. He told the authors he actually warned other rabbis he approached to join the panel that if the rabbis did not intervene, "this [case] is going to stay by the DA until the DA's decision."

The rabbis worked at a pace Rottenberg described as "emergency." And by the first week in March, even before the rabbinic court had offi-cially handed down its judgment, they were prepared to visit the DA's office, together with Hafner's attorney Jack Litman, with "new evidence" of Hafner's innocence. According to Rottenberg, Assembly Speaker Sheldon Silver, also an Orthodox Jew himself, weighed in with political support: "Shelly Silver said he's not taking sides," he said, "but he does want the doors opened [at the DA's office] to listen to what we have to say." (Silver himself did not return calls for comment.)

The critical meeting with prosecutors took place in mid-March. A few days later, the DA's office issued a statement unequivocally exonerating Rabbi Hafner. The DA's statement offered no specifics to explain its action, and its officials have never divulged details of the evidence of Hafner's innocence they are supposed to have received. Remarkably, according to the members of the rabbinic court themselves, no witnesses to any of the "evidence" in Hafner's favor ever met with the prosecutors. Rabbi Moshe Farkas, a Brooklyn rabbi, and the most active member of the court in its evidence-gathering stages, told the authors that he alone presented Bobov's case, aided only by Hafner's lawyer, to Chief Assistant District Attorney (ADA) Albert Teichman, Sex Crimes Unit head Rhonnie

Jaus, and ADA Deanne Puccio. Rabbi Rottenberg seconded Farkas's claim that no witnesses spoke to DA officials. He said that he and another member of the rabbinic panel tried to introduce community witnesses to prosecutors before Farkas's visit (and Silver's call), but "they didn't let us in the door." Attorney Litman insisted that witnesses were "presented" to DA officials, though he would not say who they were. If no witnesses were actually interviewed by prosecutors, according to Karen Burstein, a former judge, the DA's office should have required "independent confirmation" of what Farkas said. "I think if I were the DA," said Burstein, "I would be chary of acting solely on their [the rabbis'] representation."

Nor does the rabbis' evidence of Hafner's innocence appear "overwhelming," though that is how DA spokesman Davitt characterized it to the authors. According to Attorney Litman, the rabbis had discovered that the boy claimed to have been sexually abused in a place "observable by dozens and dozens of people every single day." Rottenberg explained by saying the small synagogue had "big, huge half wall windows . . . open to the street," and insisted, "There are close to a hundred people who have the combination if it would be locked. There are twenty, thirty in and out daily . . . There's a side door which everybody knows. It's open always."

But Rabbi Hafner's wife presented a different picture of the place her husband tutored the Abraham boy stating, "[The Abrahams] had asked him to learn privately [with the boy] in a very secluded place because he has a hearing aid and his hearing aid will pick up any outside noise, so he must have a quiet place. . . . He [Rabbi Hafner] tutored the child for eighteen months, once a day, in the mornings between eight and nine, *there was nobody there. . . .*"

A weekday morning visit to the site by the authors confirmed Mrs. Hafner's description. The aging Voydislaver Synagogue, a converted house, had no windows on the street level. All doors were locked and only someone standing on a ladder could have seen into the synagogue on the main floor. Through a small diamond-shaped pane in one of its three weather-beaten doors (not the main one), only a staircase leading up was dimly visible. When a buzzer next to the door was pressed, a woman's voice confirmed that the synagogue was closed, and that there were no prayers inside except on the Sabbath. No one entered or left the building between eight and nine o'clock, the time period when Hafner tutored the Abraham boy.

Mrs. Abraham said that some of Hafner's defenders simply fabricated the rabbis' details. "They had somebody go to the yeshiva down the block," she told the authors, "and tell the kids the combination [to the front door lock], so they could say a hundred people had the combination." Against this background, Ms. Burstein, the former judge, questioned the evidentiary worth of the rabbis' claim to the DA that the synagogue was wide open to the public. "'Everybody could see' requires you to show that somebody did see" what transpired between Hafner and the boy, she said. Yet no one claimed that a specific witness actually observed Hafner tutoring the child.

Besides, the rabbis seem to have made only perfunctory efforts to ascertain the mental state of the alleged child victim. Two mental health professionals were consulted by the rabbis, but neither of them interviewed the child. Toward the end of the trial, the rabbis engaged the services of Sylvan Schaffer, an Orthodox psychologist and lawyer, who is the clinical coordinator and director of education of the forensic psychiatry program at North Shore University Hospital. But remarkably, even Dr. Schaffer was not asked to interview the boy. Instead, Rottenberg claimed the rabbis merely had him interview Rabbi Hafner, plus a "random" sample of six of Hafner's other students, for any evidence that *they* had been abused.

The sketchiness of this evidence did not prevent some members of the rabbinic court from casting aspersions on the boy. "Because he's hearing impaired," said Farkas, "he always wants to get attention." Rottenberg elaborated, "The kid was bragging on and on . . . 'I want to talk more, I have more to say, I want to talk.' The child spoke for a couple of hours, begging us to listen to him more and more . . . just eating the attention with such appetite."

Nor did the rabbis pay much regard to the professionals who had supported his charges. Dr. Grimm was not invited to testify. "It was too dangerous a game, couldn't afford to lose, if you know what I mean," explained a friend of Rabbi Rottenberg who was himself a rabbi in Monsey and who made a point of referring to the Abraham boy as "the rascal." "They [the rabbis] felt a *goy* would not have the perception . . . that's the reason why this lady wasn't called."

Rottenberg himself stated he "cornered" one of the social workers who supported the boy by confronting him with the boy's claim that Rabbi Hafner had pulled his pubic hairs: "I said to him [the social worker], 'How stupid could you be?'" he remembered afterward. "A boy that age, either he doesn't have, or it's not big enough [to pull]." But Dr. Grimm told the authors that a physical examination showed the boy did have pubic hair and stated, "you don't need much" to pull it painfully. Detective Springer, though interviewed by a rabbinic court member, was, like

Dr. Grimm, not invited to testify. "There seem to be real deficiencies," said Ms. Burstein of the rabbis' handling of the case. "Not hearing testimony from a forensic specialist who examined the child . . . is troubling."

The rabbis' priorities may perhaps be gauged by Rottenberg's statement that the rabbinic court started to make tape recordings of its sessions—but stopped midway, "because they [DA officials] were going to subpoena it" and the rabbis did not believe details of child abuse allegations among Hasidim should be heard by non-Jewish authorities. And then there is Rottenberg's claim that speech pathologist Adele Markwitz, though she visited the site of the trial to offer her testimony, was kept out because she had talked about the case on WNBC television news: "Making a statement in public about a private, *innocent* person," he told the authors, "that's being low." Markwitz, who is Jewish, claimed the rabbis also said that her willingness to discuss the case publicly proved "she hates Jews."

By the time of Farkas's meeting with prosecutors, the rabbinic court had already reached its verdict. According to Rottenberg, prosecutors asked the rabbis "unofficially" not to publish their verdict before the DA's office announced its own decision to drop charges, because "they didn't want it to look like they bent under pressure." Mrs. Abraham, by contrast, had no advance warning of the outcome and was distraught when she heard it.

"'How am I gonna (sic) tell my son now that the rabbis feel he's lying?'" Rabbi Rottenberg recalled her saying. Raising his voice an octave to imitate the mother, he quoted her, "'I told him [her son] the rabbis are going to take care of Rabbi Hafner. They're going to put him into jail, punish him, and now what?' She started to go wild, claiming the *beth din* was biased, the *beth din* was all one sided . . . [She said,] 'Now our name is going to be ruined.'"

Then it was the boy's turn to get the news. Rottenberg told him, "Are you aware that we can't buy this?" He told the authors that the child answered, "But that's how it happened. It's true.'"

Community Attitudes and Reactions

There were no questions in Bobov about the rightness of the DA's decision to drop the charges. Indeed, the news spread through the Brooklyn community on March 21, 2000, a date that coincided that year with the Jewish holiday of Purim, when Jews celebrate their deliverance from threatened annihilation under ancient Persian rule. The Hasidim saw the timing of Hafner's exoneration as the work of divine providence. "By us *yidden* [Jews], we don't have the word 'coincidence' in our language," said Rottenberg. "We knew two or three days beforehand [that the charges would be dropped]. . . . In Bobov, they sang all of Purim, and Shabbos after, a *niggun* [special song] to his favor and against the [Abrahams] in a *shul* of three thousand people, the main Bobov shul. . . . Everybody knew who they meant."

Mrs. Abraham still believes Hafner is a danger to other children—and has been for years. "The only people I don't forgive in this whole story is the [other] mothers," she told the authors bitterly, "who . . . hid their heads under the rug and they kept quiet about it . . . and that's why my son got hurt, because they were selfish."

As we noted at the outset, "keeping quiet" is certainly not unheard of in ultra-Orthodox communities. Nor is a "pressure campaign" to suppress testimony by potential witnesses. In this case, the threatening notice quoted earlier in our essay was prominently displayed in a local Yiddish newspaper, signed by 50 rabbis, reminding everyone familiar with the case (that is, the entire ultra-Orthodox community of Brooklyn) that "informing" to the police was a capital crime. Hand in hand with this attitude, as part of the same sociological pattern, one continues to encounter outright denial about the reality of CSA by rabbis in the Orthodox community. A prominent rabbi well aware of this very case told the authors that "there is no problem in our community of child sexual abuse by rabbis," adding that Orthodox Jews would never face the scandal weathered by the Catholic Church because the rabbinate does not contain homosexuals.

Against this background, it is not surprising that no one in the Abrahams' community would come forward to criticize the *beth din*'s actions. In fact, once Hafner was free of the charges, even Mrs. Abraham's erstwhile supporters in the Orthodox community proved unwilling to speak publicly about the case. Rabbi Dovid Cohen, who approved the use of secular authorities, was described to the authors by a close acquaintance of his as "shell-shocked" by community criticism. Mrs. Abraham said that Cohen told her, "Let's let it die down. . . . They have a lot more political clout than we do. . . . You have to cut your losses at a certain point." Under pressure from the rabbis on the court, Cohen even wrote an open letter, which appeared on community bulletin boards, apologizing to Hafner for causing him "distress and humiliation," while nevertheless stressing his own "good intentions."

The only voices heard loudly in ultra-Orthodox circles were pro-Hafner. A month after clearing the rabbi, the five-member rabbinic court met again to issue an unusual written "blessing" to Rabbi Hafner, declaring that the charges against him were "false and based on falsehood," and asking God to compensate him for any losses incurred through his involvement in the legal system. "After all," said Rottenberg, "Rabbi Hafner has to marry off his children." Nevertheless, Henna White, Hynes's liaison to the Orthodox community, claimed to the authors that she had heard about the Hafner case everywhere she went, adding that she hoped the Abrahams's willingness to pursue their son's charges would "change things."

"She's full of baloney, in my opinion," retorted Mrs. Abraham. She and her family, after being publicly humiliated in the main Bobov synagogue where thousands sang in support of Hafner and against the Abrahams, have moved out of Brooklyn altogether. "The man will strike again. And when he strikes again, and somebody else gets hurt, that's when it will hit them."

RECOMMENDATIONS FOR NEEDED CHANGE

The example explored in this article illustrates how a religious community, driven by a set of social mores that inform the actions of that community, responded to a serious allegation of CSA by a member of its clergy. In this case, the Orthodox Jewish community vilified the alleged victim's family for turning to the secular authorities and did not appear to thoroughly investigate the allegation. What are the best ways to prevent such cases from occurring in the future?

One cannot quickly rid a community of mores formed over centuries by a complex mix of religion, sociopolitical history, and deeply ingrained memories of oppression. Anti-Semitism is still present in America, and it will be a long time before traditionally minded Jews can be habituated to a trustful relationship with this or any non-Jewish government. But reform is possible, both within and without Orthodox Jewish communities. In general, we propose reforms of two kinds: educational and legal.

Awareness Through Education

Already, to some extent, there is evidence that a few Orthodox communities, with rabbinic support, have begun to encourage education regarding CSA in schools and special forums. This new trend should be encouraged in several ways. Rabbi Mark Dratch (2006) has urged rabbis to lecture on abuse-related issues. If nothing else, he says, doing this breaks the communal norm of silence and empowers victims to begin speaking out. Next, the community, as a community, needs to be educated to the harm suffered by its members through the toleration of abuse. All too often, Jewish communal officials speak of the "community" as if abused children were not part of it, when in fact they can be found in every school, in every synagogue, on every neighborhood street. What is more, while Jews are acutely consciousness of the risks posed by ugly publicity, communities still need instruction in the costs incurred by silence. It must be realized, first, that today's abused children are part of the bulwark of tomorrow's community, and second, that sexual abuse causes long-term psychological and emotional damage to the victims, often leading in adulthood to eating disorders, sexual dysfunction, poor job performance, and a host of other psychological sequelae, all of which undermine the collective health of Jewish society. In addition, silence erodes public confidence in the institutions of the community, which by its inaction or worse seems to take the side of the criminal against the innocent. Finally, the tacit toleration of CSA means that Jewish communities will continue to be preyed on by pedophiles who are never reported to police.

Awareness of these things is already beginning to spread through Jewish communities, but, not surprisingly, progress is slow. At present, many Orthodox Jews express the belief that the airing of "old charges" by adults who were abused as children, even against rabbis who are still in contact with children, serves no purpose. This error can be corrected only by vigorous support for the survivors of CSA and sympathy for their needs. Clearly, education is needed to spur such a development.

It is also important for concerned rabbis and Jewish communal leaders to become acquainted with and to circulate the growing literature on Jewish law that supports the needs of abuse victims. This can be done by insisting on the duty to report abuse to police or other authorities, defending the right of victims to speak the truth, and placing the blame for "desecration of God's name" through adverse publicity squarely on the abusers where it belongs. Our experience suggests that few religious Jews are aware that such rulings exist. If local rabbis were to include these rulings in some of their classes and lectures, the effects could be significant.

Legal Reform

Important legal reforms must also be undertaken outside Orthodox Jewish circles. It is essential that prosecutors, journalists, and others involved in the criminal justice system speak out forcefully about any mechanism that facilitates cover-ups of clerical sexual abuse. To some extent, this simply means following existing law and policy directives, which up to now have not been sufficiently enforced. For example, New York's Executive Law, Section 642(1) specifically requires that the "victim of a violent felony offense" (which CSA is) or, where the victim is a minor, "the family of the victim . . . shall be consulted by the district attorney in order to obtain the views of the victim regarding disposition of the criminal case by dismissal." This was clearly *not* done in the Hafner case, though the offense in question was certainly a violent felony and the alleged child victim was a minor. If the law had been followed, perhaps prosecutors would have given the rabbinic court's "evidence" the second look it deserved, at a minimum.

Another way in which law enforcement authorities can rein in the overreaching of rabbinic courts in criminal cases is to apply to them the same standards and methods they are already accustomed to using when witnesses are intimidated by gangs or organized crime. We do not mean that rabbinic courts are composed of criminals, or that their methods are often the same as those of criminal gangs; however, within their communities rabbinic tactics can be just as intimidating and can undermine justice just as effectively. Therefore, secular law enforcement authorities must be educated about the potential of rabbinic courts to interfere with victims and witnesses in CSA investigations and must learn to act accordingly. Again, New York already has an applicable statute; section 641(2) of the Executive Law requires "notification of a victim or a witness as to steps that law enforcement officers or district attorneys can take to protect victims and witnesses from intimidation." There is simply no evidence that this statute has ever been applied to the Orthodox Jewish community. As the example of the case discussed here shows, in which the parents were allegedly pressured by the rabbinic court to recant their charges, it should be.

The legal system is part of a society's web of governing institutions, and it is critical that everyone connected with it recognize the importance of enforcing the laws against CSA everywhere, including inside religious Jewish communities. Prosecutors must both liaison effectively with a community whose norms may be somewhat foreign to them and, at the same time, stand aloof from improper influence. Perhaps no prosecutors can completely ignore the significance of large voting blocs, but they can establish policies that, for example, bar prosecutors from relying on religious courts to take over their function. Such a practice, so central to the

Hafner case, raises serious constitutional questions. The general public can and should demand that all abused children be given the same sort of treatment in the criminal justice system. Journalists, too, must do their part, informing the public about the miscarriages of justice caused by rabbinic interference and the failure of law enforcement officials to apply their own laws to such cases.

CONCLUSION

The authors of this article are themselves Orthodox Jews, and do not regard their argument as an attack on Jewish tradition. Rather, they urge a healthy examination and maturation of the community's social mores, which have not yet come to grips with the modern-day needs of children sexually abused by rabbis. As the eminent critic Hugh Kenner (1959) commented in an analysis of the role of the past in shaping the present:

> . . . Tradition is not a bin into which you relegate what you cannot be bothered to examine, but precisely that portion of the past . . . which you have examined scrupulously. You cannot admire, you cannot learn from, you cannot even rebel against what you do not know. (p. 117)

The spread of knowledge and understanding about CSA committed by rabbis, and the tactics by which these offenses have been concealed, can only help to produce a saner and healthier future in traditional Jewish communities. And no one in the Orthodox or non-Orthodox world is likely to deny that we are at precisely that juncture in modern Jewish history.

NOTES

1. Nearly all Orthodox Jews send their children to private schools where religious education is an important part of the curriculum. The more traditional of such schools are called *yeshivas*; where religious discipline is less strict, such schools are usually known as "day schools."

2. Within this and the following two sections, "Intervention of the *Beth Din*" and "Community Attitudes and Reactions," there are more than 25 quotations drawn from personal communications. These quotations were drawn from face-to-face interviews, phone conversations, and e-mails. For the purposes of readability, each of these quotations will not be cited individually as a personal communication.

REFERENCES

Ain, S. (1990, August 24). Sex abuse suspect charged in fraud case. *The Jewish Week, 7.*

Babylonian Talmud, *Baba Kamma* 116b–117a, *Gittin* 7a.

Dratch, M. (1992, April). Published proceedings of the Rabbinic Council of America Roundtable, pp. 1–18.

Dratch, M. (2006, January 19). Domestic abuse is a community issue. Retrieved September 4, 2007, from www.JSafe.org/pdfs/community%20issue.pdf

Glick, M. (2000, February 4). Dealing with "Orthodox" child molesters: A response to the community's response [Letter to the editor]. *The Jewish Press*, 87–88.

Kenner, H. (1959). *The invisible poet: T. S. Eliot.* New York: McDowell, Obolensky.

Kings County District Attorney's Office. (2000, March 20). Statement from the Kings County District Attorney's Office regarding Solomon Hafner. Public release. Brooklyn, NY: Kings County District Attorney's Office.

Neusner, J. (1970). Rabbis and community in third century Babylonia. In J. Neusner (Ed.), *Religions in antiquity* (pp. 438–459). Leiden: E. J. Brill.

"Notice." (2000, June 8). *Der Blatt*, p. 8.

The rebbes: The Lubavitcher Rebbe Shlita. (Translation from Hebrew). (1993). Kfar Chabad: Chish Printing Co.

Rosenbluth, S. (2006, July). Abuse in the Orthodox community and the *Beit Din. The Jewish Voice and Opinion*, pp. 11–21.

Shulhan Arukh, Hoshen ha-Mishpat 388:9.

Winerip, M. (1994, February 4). Yeshivas wield political power. *New York Times*, p. A16.

The Impact of the Clergy Abuse Scandal on Parish Communities

Paul M. Kline
Robert McMackin
Edna Lezotte

The Archdiocese of Boston has been at the center of the clergy sexual abuse crisis in the Roman Catholic Church. Since the scandal exploded into public awareness in late 2002, Boston's Catholic community has witnessed agonizing testimony from hundreds of victims. During 2003, firsthand accounts of betrayal and abuse by Catholic clergy were reported by news outlets almost weekly. Additionally, the legal discovery process as well as the work of investigative journalists uncovered documents verifying that priest perpetrators were intentionally transferred among parishes by church hierarchy at the expense of children, their families, and parish communities. In 2003, Boston's Catholics also witnessed the resignation of their cardinal, Bernard Law, whose credibility as a moral and spiritual leader was damaged beyond repair by the central role he played in the church's mismanagement of the problem.

The crisis in Boston has involved an unexpected, overwhelming, and inescapable flood of disturbing disclosures of sexual crimes against children by esteemed members of an "honored class" (Rubin, 2004). The abusive behavior was not isolated to a few members of the "honored class," but reached into the highest levels of the ecclesial structure to implicate, through collusion and inaction, numerous bishops. The criminal misconduct of perpetrator-priests combined with the betrayal of the laity by church leaders posed a threat to the spiritual and psychosocial well-being of faith communities in Boston. This was additionally complicated by the financial settlement with more than 500 victims, which strained the Archdiocese of Boston's financial resources.

Although many people first became aware of the clergy sexual abuse scandal as a Boston crisis, it soon became painfully obvious that the problem touched every diocese in the United States. A study authorized by the United States Conference of Catholic Bishops (United States Conference of Catholic Bishops, 2005) acknowledged that "the sexual abuse of children and young people . . . and the ways in which these crimes and sins were addressed, have caused enormous pain, anger, and confusion" (Preamble, para 1). This same study documented that between 1950 and 2002 more than 10,000 boys and girls had been abused by Catholic clergy. It noted that this abuse was not isolated to particular archdioceses but was a pervasive pattern found throughout the United States. This pattern of abuse by Catholic clergy has led to numerous civil and criminal lawsuits. Five archdioceses have formally declared bankruptcy and others are at risk of bankruptcy. The profound impact of these events on the American Catholic Church, in respect to its moral leadership, spiritual direction, and fiscal stability, can hardly be overestimated. This article offers a discussion of the impact caused by this catastrophic crisis for practicing Catholic adults who are not primary victims of clergy sexual abuse.

PARISH FOCUS GROUPS

In 2003, the "Church in the 21st Century" initiative at Boston College awarded a grant to faculty members from the Boston College Graduate School of Social Work and practitioners from the Boston Archdiocesan Office of Pastoral Support and Outreach. The overarching purpose of the grant was to develop and pilot a group intervention to assist secondary victims of clergy sexual abuse. Secondary victims were considered those who were not directly abused by clergy or members of their immediate family, including parents, siblings, or spouses.

As part of the grant planning process, three focus groups were held in parishes that had been directly impacted by clergy sexual abuse. Parishes where the current pastor had expressed support for the goal of the initiative and one or more perpetrator-priests had been previously stationed were selected as focus group sites.

Drawing on the pastor's knowledge of the parish community and with the assistance of other parish leaders, groups were populated with voluntary participants whose involvement in parish life ranged from minimal to very active. Since the intervention was targeted at nonabused adult Catholics, individuals with a personal history of clergy abuse or who knew of a family member who had been abused by a priest were not included in a focus group. Group members were required to keep the names of participants confidential and were promised that public discussion of what was learned from the focus groups would not be attached to a specific individual by name or to a specific parish community. All of the participants gave permission for the team to prepare a written summary from the focus groups, without identifying participants by name, for the purpose of assisting the Boston Archdiocese as well as other Catholic communities in responding to the clergy abuse scandal.

Twenty-four adults (6 men and 18 women) participated in the focus groups. Although participants were not asked to provide personal demographic data, information disclosed during the course of group sessions strongly suggests that nearly all participants were registered, active members of a specific parish in the Archdiocese of Boston. Focus group sessions lasted two hours and all three groups were lead by the same two mental health professionals. A third team member recorded a verbatim transcript of all group sessions.

Participants were invited to respond to the following questions: (a) What disturbs you most about the revelations regarding the clergy abuse scandal? (b) How have your reactions to the disclosures of abuse changed over time? (c) Have the disclosures of abuse altered your relationship with God? (d) Have the disclosures of abuse altered your relationship with the church? (e) Does your parish need anything for healing or reconciliation? (f) How do you think the church should reach out to those who have been alienated from the church due to the scandal?

Each group lasted the full two hours and the meetings were often emotionally charged. Many participants became noticeably upset during the course of the discussions. All group members were provided access to a mental health professional in the days and weeks after the group session as a resource for coping with any unexpected or disturbing reactions to the focus group experience. None of the participants made use of this supportive resource.

Participants initially expressed strong anger at perpetrator-priests. Some were disturbed at having discovered that they had once received sacraments from priests who were now accused or convicted of sexual crimes against children. Once the culpability of perpetrator-priests was acknowledged and participants' anger at those priests discharged, participants turned attention to their urgent and powerful need to express thoughts and very strong feelings about the role played by church leaders in the clergy sexual abuse scandal. Four major themes, common to all groups and shared by most participants, were clearly identified and are discussed.

Deep Hurt in Response to a Perceived Betrayal by Church Leaders

The Catholic men and women who participated in these focus groups were deeply hurt by the many "discoveries" that, together, make up this complex scandal. Consequently, they might appropriately be considered as "secondary victims" of clergy abuse (Hopkins, 1991; Rubin, 2004). Similar to Doyle's (2003) observations about direct victims of abuse, we observed that nonabused adults directed their "deepest and most abiding sense of anger and frustration . . . toward the ecclesiastical leadership: bishops, religious superiors and the pope" (p. 204–205). Some participants expressed a belief that there was no meaningful moral difference between the criminal actions of perpetrator-priests and the behavior of church leaders. Powerful emotions of despair, anger, and bitterness surfaced as they described church leaders as "deceitful," "arrogant," and "hypocritical." Participants reported having reached the firm conclusion that church leaders were guilty of violating a "sacred trust" with the faithful. Many believed that this betrayal caused a rupture in the relationship between bishops and the laity, and described their parish community as operating with no strong feeling of being "connected" with the archdiocesan hierarchy. Furthermore, participants shared a concern that the rupture in the relationship between "the people" and bishops and cardinals might never be repaired.

Perhaps more significantly, this rupture was also experienced by many at a very private level. Participants reported that their personal, emotional connection to church leadership was now severely damaged. Anguish and grief surfaced as they described this damage to their affective attachment to church leaders. The powerful emotions of anger and resentment seemed, in part, to be a reaction to the loss of a warm connection to their bishop. Discussion of this important experience revealed that, for many, the rupture in the emotional connection to church leaders occurred in response to what participants perceived as the true motives behind church leaders' improper decisions when confronted by the problem of clergy sexual abuse of minors. The decisions to transfer accused priests, to encourage silence from victims and their families, and to avoid criminal prosecution of those accused of serious crimes against children were interpreted by most participants as a manifestation of indifference or even contempt for the faithful on the part of church leaders. Consequently, the attachment that participants once experienced as grounded in authentic concern, devotion, respect, and love (Plante, 2004; Rossetti, 1997) was reinterpreted as rooted in an administrative culture of ruthlessness and exploitation. In response to this "discovery," participants described strong feelings of "disgust" toward bishops and cardinals as well as a burden of personal shame. Many described their church as now "stained" and "soiled." These observations are supported by recent research suggesting that in response to the uncovering of sexual abuse by Catholic clergy, "feelings of shame and embarrassment are widely shared by both registered parishioners and other Catholics" (Davidson & Hoge, 2004, p. 15).

A Reawakening of Pain Connected to Past Injuries by the Church

Learning about the terrible history of clergy abuse of children and the failure of church leaders to protect children, families, and parish communities caused some participants to revisit and reinterpret their difficult past experiences with priests and with the institutional church. Many described having become preoccupied with memories of past moments in time when they experienced a priest or other church representative as insensitive to their needs or as unkind in responding to their concerns. These recollections included accounts of priests refusing to preside at marriages or funerals and being insensitive at a time of crisis, such as ascribing an illness to a person's sinful behavior. These memories came alive in the groups with surprising clarity and power and were often accompanied by strong feelings of bitterness. They were frequently presented as moments in time when participants felt misunderstood and judged harshly, producing feelings of embarrassment or shame. These unpleasant encounters, occurring at an earlier time in a participant's life, appeared to have been reexamined and filtered through the emotional and cognitive changes connected to the current clergy abuse crisis. These past hurts were now understood as having been "caused" by the same indifference and contempt on the part of church leaders that participants believed to be a major factor in the perpetuation of the clergy abuse scandal. This finding is consistent with Steinfels's (2002) suggestion that Catholics may now be struggling to cope with "the cumulative effect of years of irritations with what looks like the indifference, incompetence, or arrogance of church leaders" (p. 18).

The Separation of Relationship with God from Relationship with the Church

The clergy abuse scandal in the Catholic Church can be understood as a complicated and overwhelming event that, for some, has disturbed and disrupted core religious beliefs and familiar patterns of religious practice (Falsetti, Resick & Davis, 2003). The damaged relationship with church leaders described previously is one symptom of such a disturbance. In addition, in every group a sharp distinction was drawn by participants between their current relationship with God and their current relationship with "the church." Even as participants reported a more distant and conflicted relationship to church leaders, many also described a "stronger relationship" with God. Although most reported continued, regular participation in the sacraments, some made a sharp distinction between their participation "on the outside" and their "internal" experience. The new interior experience seemed to involve a different emotional connection to the priest. Participants reported that their devotion to the sacraments involved an altered emotional investment, with their focal point being the sacramental act rather than the priest presiding at the ritual. These descriptions suggested that some participants experienced the "person" of the priest to be a distraction. Some intentionally avoided watching the priest perform sacred rituals so as to avoid being reminded about the scandalous behavior of other priests. This depersonalizing of the priest might be understood as a consequence of the priest serving as the "official representative of the Church" (Compliment, 1998, p. 12). Catholics may now express their anger at church leaders through an altered relationship to priests. Perhaps, too, the crisis has conditioned parishioners to see all priests as tainted by the criminal misconduct of perpetrators. Many participants expressed sad resignation that no new allegation of misconduct against *any* priest or church leader could now "surprise" or "shock" them. This may reveal the unfortunate spread of anger and mistrust for those responsible for the scandal to other priests and bishops.

Compliment (1998) has noted that "the closer one is to actual knowledge of clergy misconduct, the less likely it is one will remain satisfied with the quality of priests in the Church" (p. 92). Focus groups participants could accurately be described as burdened with detailed knowledge of clergy misconduct in their parishes and in their archdiocese. In spite of the noteworthy sorrow, grief, and anger expressed by participants, many also reported finding new means of spiritual sustenance such as journaling, meditation, walking in a nature preserve, and intimacy with friends. Some indicated that their dissatisfaction with priests and church hierarchy led to their seeking a relationship with God in new ways. These expressions of a stronger personal spirituality were seen by most as positive adaptations to the crisis. The dedication to preserving a relationship with God may be seen as an indicator of the importance of personal spiritual health for these participants. However, participants' report of increased separation between their personal relationship with God and their relationship to their church poses a significant challenge as well. A long-term coping strategy that remains rooted in a pervasive mistrust of priests and church leadership may contribute to erosion in the spiritual vitality of the parish community that, in time, threatens the spiritual well-being of all community members.

A Concern for the Spiritual Well-Being of Children and Family

Most participants expressed strong confidence in their relationship with God and, despite experiencing a dramatic change in their emotional connection to priests and to church leaders, most predicted that they would continue to actively practice their faith. However, many described high levels of concern for the spiritual well-being of close family members—especially spouses and children. Intense sorrow accompanied stories of family members having withdrawn from all involvement in the sacraments and from the local parish community. Descriptions of angry outbursts by spouses and by adolescent and adult children, some promising to "never" return to the church, were common. Many of these practicing Catholics were now members of families that no longer worshiped together, and some offered descriptions of families that had lost their shared Catholic identity.

These stories are noteworthy for several reasons. They suggest that the steady presence of a parent or spouse who remains committed to their Catholic faith may not be enough to sustain the faith of close family members whose anger and pain in response to the scandal is strong. While many of the participants in these groups remained devoted to their Catholic spirituality, they experienced acute despair that those closest to them were now "out of reach." Participants expressed hope that the Boston Archdiocese would openly address the situation and provide assistance in responding to the hostile withdrawal of their loved ones from the church.

Anticipating that family members might be forever lost to the church, some participants demonstrated anticipatory grief over future family events (births, deaths, marriages) that, they now believed, would be compromised by the absence of a sacramental experience. As these participants looked into their family's future, some predicted that the toxic effects of the clergy abuse scandal would ripple out to negatively affect future events in the life of their family. This grief added another layer of suffering to the challenge of coping with the clergy abuse scandal and may represent an ongoing threat to the spiritual well-being of those struggling to remain connected to their faith and church. Friberg (1995) has noted that the loss of religious experience at individual and family "life-marking events" as a consequence of clergy sexual misconduct can produce a "feeling of personal and spiritual betrayal or treason" (p. 58). Also, within the same family some members may cope with this betrayal by envisioning a future where important family events are free from the stain of the church's involvement while other family members long for the moment to be marked by traditional religious practice. Some participants feared that conflicts between family members would be long-term and worried that no healthy resolution would be possible.

CONCLUSION

The clergy abuse crisis in the Catholic Church has been described as "a continuing failure to respect the basic human dignity of the individual victims, their families, the potential victims, and the community at large" (Rubin, 2004, p. 81). A recent survey by Davidson and Hoge (2004) indicated that American Catholics identify this as the most serious issue facing the church and that "both the personal and institutional facets of the scandal are considered serious" (p. 14).

On a personal level, many Catholics have discovered that some priests, who were a meaningful part of the story of their lives, were simultaneously engaged in criminal acts of sexual violence against minors. This discovery causes them to question the "legitimacy" of sacred moments involving those priests. Places of worship that at one time offered comfort and peace may now be experienced as having been soiled. New encounters with good priests are filtered through the prism of clergy pedophilia, resulting in a formal and emotionally distant relationship with a pastor or parish priest. Some priests, acutely aware of these doubts and suspicions on the part of their parishioners and anticipating hostility or rejection, may respond to this emotional withdrawal by assuming a more safe and distant emotional posture. As a result, a widening gulf between priests and parishioners threatens the spiritual and psychosocial benefits that are realized through a full involvement with others in a faith community.

Finally, for some Catholics the clergy abuse scandal has disrupted long-standing patterns of family and community worship, causing division and conflict. In the wake of this tension, some are burdened with grief and despair over the loss of cherished traditions through which a family affirms its shared devotion and faith through religious ritual. Given the complex and deep personal impact of the clergy abuse crisis, it would not seem unreasonable to worry that, for some Catholics, "the scandal . . . poisons the very integrity of the Catholic identity" (O'Brien, 2003, p. 14–15).

Rossetti (1997) has suggested that strong leadership, clear information, and swift action in response to credible allegations are needed to address the erosion of trust between Catholics and their bishops and priests. Testimony from participants in these focus groups suggested that these steps are necessary to restore confidence in the church's capacity to make better decisions when confronted with allegations of priestly misconduct. However, many participants indicated that their worry about the capacity of church leaders to change policies was reinforced by their belief that their bishops and cardinals "simply do not care," as evidenced by their prior responses to allegations of clergy-perpetrated sexual abuse.

Church leaders must respond to the laity's knowledge that cardinals and bishops failed to honor their promise to love and care for the faithful if they hope to fully address the impact of clergy sexual abuse. Although comforted by a strong connection to God, many Catholics have experienced a dramatic and painful change in their affective connection to their church leaders. The clergy abuse scandal has been interpreted by many as strong evidence that bishops, cardinals, and priests are incapable of authentic and enduring feelings of love, concern, and empathy. Priests and bishops eager to reengage the laity in a relationship of goodwill and trust may be surprised by the strength of the laity's "resistance" to "forgiving" church leaders. The hurt associated with the discovery that a promise of love and protection was a lie can produce remarkably deep layers of self-protection from future betrayal. The USCCB has expressed an awareness of the rupture in their relationship with those they have promised to serve. Hopefully, they will find meaningful and effective ways to honor their pledge to "recommit . . . to a continual pastoral outreach to repair the breach with those who have suffered sexual abuse and with all of the people of the Church" (United States Conference of Catholic Bishops, 2005, Preamble, para 19).

REFERENCES

Compliment, B. K. (1998). The other victims of scandal in the church: A study of the effects of clergy misconduct on ministerial identity, coping response and style of faith development of non-offending priests and laity in the Roman Catholic church. *Dissertation Abstracts International, 58*(8-B), 1–485.

Davidson, J. D., & Hoge, D. R. (2004). Catholics after the scandal: A new study's major findings. *Commonweal, 131*, 13–19.

Doyle, T. P. (2003). Roman Catholic clericalism, religious duress, and clergy sexual abuse. *Pastoral Psychology, 51*, 189–231.

Falsetti, S. A., Resick, P. A., & Davis, J. L. (2003). Changes in religious beliefs following trauma. *Journal of Traumatic Stress, 16*, 391–398.

Friberg, N. (1995). Wounded congregations. In N. M. Hopkins & M. Laaser (Eds.), *Restoring the soul of a church* (pp. 55–76). Collegeville, MN: The Liturgical Press.

Hopkins, N. (1991). Congregational intervention when the pastor has committed sexual misconduct. *Pastoral Psychology, 39,* 247–255.

O'Brien, D. (2003). How to solve the church crisis: Ordinary Catholics must act. *Commonweal, 130,* 10–15.

Plante, T. G. (2004). Bishops behaving badly: Ethical considerations regarding the clergy abuse crisis in the Roman Catholic Church. *Ethics & Human Behavior, 14,* 67–87.

Rossetti, S. J. (1997). The effects of priest-perpetration of child sexual abuse on the trust of Catholics in the priesthood, Church, and God. *Journal of Psychology and Christianity, 16,* 197–209.

Rubin. S. S. (2004). Why was I not my brother's keeper—Or my own? *Ethics & Human Behavior, 14,* 77–82.

Steinfels, P. (2002). The church's sex-abuse crisis: What's old, what's new, what's needed now. *Commonweal, 12,* 13–19.

United States Conference of Catholic Bishops, Office for the Protection of Children and Young People. (2005). *Charter for the protection of children and young people.* Retrieved November 6, 2006, from http://www.usccb.org/ocyp/charter.shtml.

THEORETICAL CONSIDERATIONS

A Theoretical Foundation for Understanding Clergy-Perpetrated Sexual Abuse

Jason M. Fogler
Jillian C. Shipherd
Erin Rowe
Jennifer Jensen
Stephanie Clarke

> Now in accordance with the Canons, you have been selected to serve God in [this] Church. This . . . is a sign that you are fully empowered and authorized to exercise this ministry, accepting its privileges and responsibilities as a priest of this Diocese, in communion with your Bishop. . . . Having committed yourself to this work, do not forget the trust of those who have chosen you. Care alike for young and old, strong and weak, rich and poor. (The Episcopal Church, 1979, p. 557)

Clergy-perpetrated sexual abuse (CPSA) has been deemed the "worst crisis" in the Catholic Church's American history and the late Pope John Paul II's papacy (Paulson, 2005). More than 10,000 allegations of CPSA were made by Catholic parishioners between 1950–2002, with 81% of survivors being male and more than 40% of all survivors being boys aged 11–14 (The John Jay College Research Team, 2004). The Associated Press (2005) reported that settlements between the Catholic Church and survivors have exceeded $1 billion. Although the sexual abuse crisis in the Catholic Church has received the majority of recent media attention, it is not the only Christian denomination or religious group to encounter this problem. CPSA has also been discussed in the Episcopal (Richards, 2004), Protestant (Disch & Avery, 2001; Fortune, 1989), Buddhist (Simpkinson, 1996), and Jewish faiths ("Jewish Sexual Abuse," n.d; see also Neustein & Lesher, 2008).

Efforts to understand CPSA and its effects have been largely based in qualitative interview studies of survivors (Bera, 1995; Flynn, 2000; Fortune, 1989; Isely, 1996; also see Isely, Isley, Freiburger, & McMackin, 2008; Flynn, 2008). These studies underscore links between CPSA and what is known about other forms of sexual abuse, especially the sexual abuse of children (e.g., Farrell & Taylor, 2000; Isely & Isely, 1990). CPSA and other forms of sexual abuse appear to share similar relational dynamics between survivors and perpetrators and similar psychological conse-quences, including symptoms of simple and complex post-traumatic stress disorder (PTSD; see Herman, 1992; Kohlenberg & Tsai, 1998). It is well established that sexual abuse can have long-term negative consequences, including chronic depression, self-destructive behavior, isolation, damaged sense of self-esteem and trust in others, substance abuse, anxiety, anger, and aggression (Allers, Benjack, & Allers 1992; Gagnon & Hersen, 2000). In addition to the similarities with other forms of abuse, Farrell and Taylor (2000) and McLaughlin (1994) noted that symptoms of spiritual and theo-logical crisis during and after the abuse set CPSA apart from other forms of sexual abuse and therefore advocated that it be studied as a separate entity.

Having a theoretical foundation for understanding CPSA is the first step toward developing and testing effective interventions for survivors, perpetrators, and religious communities. We are not the first to make this argument. A special issue of *Studies in Gender and Sexuality* (Frawley O'Dea & Goldner, 2004) was devoted to analyzing the problem of CPSA from a theoretical perspective, and a growing number of writers have strongly advocated for methodologically rigorous work in this area (e.g., McGlone, 2003). Unfortunately, no comprehensive theoretical framework exists for understanding the complex set of interrelationships between perpe-trators, survivors, and their communities. We propose to review some possi-ble ways of conceptualizing the phenomenon of CPSA. We seek to stimulate future hypothesis-driven clinical research into CPSA by providing a discus-sion of a few applicable (and we believe, testable) theoretical models derived from research into other forms of sexual abuse, as well as CPSA.

OVERVIEW AND DISCLAIMER

From our review of the literature, we believe that CPSA and its psy-chological consequences can best be conceptualized as an *interactive dynamic process* between perpetrators, survivors, and religious commu-nities. CPSA by definition includes a clergyperson's inappropriate sex-ual advances and behavior, but it also includes the cultivation of a relationship in which these behaviors occur, the theological and community context surrounding this usually secret and forbidden relationship, and the impact and psychological aftershock of abusive behavior on the survivor and community. These relational processes have direct and delayed effects that are not easily analyzed in aggregate but can be studied at the individual or subgroup level. By reducing the model into smaller, more testable parts, the complexity of CPSA can begin to be explored.

As an interactive dynamic process, CPSA includes three broad, over-lapping thematic categories: (a) the abusive relationship between the perpetrator and the survivor, (b) the relationship between the survivor and the larger community upon disclosure of the abuse, and (c) the relation-ship between the clergyperson and the community once the clergyperson has been identified as an alleged perpetrator. This view is congruent with Goldner's (2004) conceptualization of CPSA as a story told from the perspectives of the victim/survivor, the professional/clergy, and the "bystander" (family member, community, etc.), but we attempt to go one step further by highlighting what could be empirically studied mechanisms and inferred "cause-effect" relationships within this fluid, interactive narrative. These mechanisms are derived from the existing literature on sexual abuse more generally, and we hope to create a base on which a theory of CPSA can be built that also highlights some of the unique aspects of this traumatic experience. From this point forward, we will refer to the three core interactive processes as themes and discuss the mechanisms we believe are present in each core theme. Additionally, we realize the perpetrator in CPSA can be either a man or woman from any faith orientation, yet for this paper we will generally refer to the clergy perpetrator as a "clergyman" as the predomi-nant number of cases of CPSA involves men as the perpetrators.

We acknowledge that our discussion is a biased one in that we have chosen a selection of theoretical elements that fit our conceptual prejudices. For example, we draw heavily from Summit's (1983) writing about the Child Sexual Abuse Accommodation Syndrome (CSAAS), which addresses the question of what dynamics trap children in sexually abusive relation-ships, and Isely and Isely's (1990) application of Summit's model to CPSA in adult survivors. Such broadly inclusive models are appealing in that they discuss dynamics that we believe are applicable to both child and adult survivors of CPSA. We focus in particular on the clergyman's direct abuse of his trusted position. We also draw from the highly influential Trauma-genic Dynamics Model (Finkelhor & Browne, 1986), which subsumes the disparate reactions of sexually traumatized children under four thematic cat-egories: (a) traumatic sexualization, (b) stigmatization, (c) betrayal, and (d) powerlessness. Each theme has three subcomponents: dynamics, psycho-logical impact, and behavioral manifestations. Not all CPSA survivors will manifest dynamics and behaviors for every theme, but the model's wide scope maximizes the likelihood of conceptualizing the survivor's behavior.

We expect that by sketching a broad but empirically informed model we will be able to capture the complexities and nuances of CPSA. However, we stress that this article is in no way intended to be the "final word" on CPSA. Rather, it is our hope that future researchers will either add to or amend our initial model as more data become available.

THEME 1: RELATIONSHIPS BETWEEN PERPETRATORS AND SURVIVORS

The first theme is represented by four primary mechanisms that shape the relationship between perpetrator and survivor. These mechanisms are: the abuse of clerical power, the use of God to leverage the abusive relationship, the relationship's impact on self-concept, and the role of predatory clergy. Each mechanism is discussed with considerations for future research.

Perpetrators and Survivors: The Abuse of Clerical Power to Sexually Exploit Others

The dynamics of sexual misconduct and abuse between helping professionals and their clients (e.g., Disch & Avery, 2001; Penfold, 1999) provides a helpful starting point. Except in extreme cases of violent rape and sexual intimidation using quid-pro-quo tactics, it can be difficult to recognize the abusive quality of sexually inappropriate relationships between clergy and adult parishioners. At first glance, some may say that these relationships have more in common with developmentally appropriate romantic relationships or affairs. For example, Francis and Turner (1995) distinguished adult women parishioners whose "admiration for a pastor develops into sexual feelings" (p. 218) as a separate category from those who seem to act out past sexual trauma or other psychopathology or who enter a sexual relationship while seeking counsel during such highly vulnerable periods as marital or other personal crises. However, the inherent power of the pastoral role has important repercussions that transcend these subdivisions of relationship. As evidence, the literature in this area suggests that many abusive dynamics are present in "consenting" adult relationships between people of unequal power. Glaser and Thorpe (1986) surveyed female psychology graduate students who entered into sexual relationships with their academic advisors and observed a statistically significant shift from an initially positive or neutral view of the relationship to a negative one over time. In addition, Penfold's (1999) qualitative study of women who were involved in sexually exploitative relationships with either a licensed medical or mental health professional or member of the clergy produced findings that were remarkably similar to findings from the previously described qualitative research on CPSA. The women in Penfold's study initially felt special to be "singled out" by the counselor for such an intimate relationship but over time felt increasingly exploited and developed clinically significant symptoms of depression, anxiety, and somatization. Thus, qualitative data demonstrate support for the hypothesis that there is an abusive quality to these relationships.

Despite the abusive quality of someone with authority and power gaining access to a survivor through their unique standing in the community, many survivors express ambivalence about filing a complaint against the abuser. To understand this situation, theoretical models such as the CSAAS (Summit, 1983) are enlightening. Dynamics such as "entrapment and accommodation" are very well described. In this dynamic, the sexually abused person internalizes a false sense of control over the abuse experiences and believes that if he or she can just learn how to be "good" in the perpetrator's eyes, the victim can reduce the abuse's frequency, if not avoid it altogether, and maybe even elicit the perpetrator's positive attention and behavior. Similarly, Simpkinson (1996) described how adult women were convinced by their Buddhist teacher that they could "only achieve enlightenment by serving the sexual and other needs of their enlightened master" (p. 3).

The abuse of power is most often discussed in cases of incest, which we believe has direct application to CPSA. For example, some Christian denominations call priests "Father," which has symbolic meaning for describing the priest's role in the community. Herman and Hirschman (1977, 1981) and others (Courtois, 1988; Goodwin, Cormier, & Owen, 1983; Russell, 1986) discuss how father-daughter, brother-sister, uncle-niece, and grandfather-granddaughter incest frequently occurs in highly patriarchal societies in which fathers have unquestioned authority. Male perpetrators of incestuous abuse often enforce their will through domestic violence and "family tyranny" (Herman, 1993). Summit (1983) wrote that when survivors are chronically overwhelmed in this manner by their perpetrators, both physically and emotionally, a common reaction is internalized helplessness. This reaction may be especially likely to occur in cases in which the perpetrator is an authority figure with whom the survivor has a close, dependent, and often isolated relationship.

Mirroring the findings related to incest, Franz (2002) and Rossetti (1995) described how sexual exploitation may be facilitated by the patriarchal structure of Christian faiths and the exalted role of priests and ministers (see also McGlone, 2003; Richards, 2004). In Christian faiths (and one could argue all of the world's dominant monotheistic religions), the pastor's leadership and love of his church and congregation are proxy for the leadership and love of God. Whether a clergyman counsels a congregant or suggests a plan for the church's growth and development, the wisdom and correctness of his decisions are understood to stem from the depth of his spiritual connection. Within this context, a survivor may believe that to deny a perpetrating clergyman's advances is to deny the wishes and moral authority of God. This basic formulation holds whether the survivor is an adult or a child. For example, Fortune (1989) compellingly wrote about the confusion of one congregant when she was approached by her pastor to enter a sexual relationship in secret:

> Was her pastor's suggestion appropriate? Was it ethical? Was it right for her? She realized that she had missed the emotional and sexual intimacy she had shared with her husband, and she longed to have that again. [She] shared her hesitation and questions with [her pastor]. *He was her pastor and she trusted and respected him.* As she wavered, [the pastor] reassured her: It was perfectly acceptable; *she should know that he would not suggest anything that was not for her well-being.* (p. 20, our emphases)

Dynamics such as traumatic sexualization, secrecy, and powerlessness highlight the discrepancy between the powerful clergyman and the less powerful adult parishioner. This dynamic could be exacerbated in the case of children. Finkelhor and Browne (1986) described how children internalize a false sense of control over abusive experiences, and children in incestuous relationships are often placed in the developmentally inappropriate role of surrogate spouse and made to feel responsible for fulfilling the abusive parent's emotional and physical needs (Courtois, 1988; Hunter, 1990). The psychological impact on the child, and we would make a similar argument in the case of adult survivors, is confusion about appropriate sexual relations and identity, aversion to sex and intimacy as a result of traumatic conditioning, and the false association between sex and caregiving/ caregetting. We discuss the perpetrating clergyman's explicit use of God to leverage sexual exploitation later in this paper, but the implicit power of the clerical role, even if it is never explicitly invoked during CPSA events, cannot be overstated.

As reviewed previously, there is strong anecdotal evidence and qualitative data to support the hypothesis that the inherent power of the clergyman's role is a salient variable in any sexual relationship with parishioners. This evidence highlights the exploitive and abusive nature of these relationships even when the survivors are adults at the time of the abuse. An important next step in this line of research is to continue to document similarities and differences between CPSA survivors and other types of survivors of exploitive relationships. For example, one new direction in this literature might be to document the patterns of symptoms that are present in CPSA survivors (e.g., PTSD) and to compare these symptoms to the symptom profiles of survivors of incest or other exploitive relationships. In this way, it will be possible to determine if recovery from CPSA, or lack thereof, follows a similar trajectory to recovery from other types of abuse of power. Similarly, it might be useful to begin to evaluate the cognitions of CPSA survivors in a systematic way to determine whether cognitions that are consistent with entrapment and accommodation are present. There are already established measures such as the Personal Beliefs and Reactions Scale (Resick, Schnicke, & Markway, 1991) that might be useful in this regard. Given that these constructs are central to some types of empirically supported psychotherapy (e.g., Cognitive Processing Therapy), we would expect that they would also be applicable to the evidence-based treatment of CPSA survivors. Moreover, measures of internalized hopelessness (e.g., Pearlin & Schooler, 1987) would be important to gather, as well as thorough evaluations of how the experience was framed by the clergyman during the abuse. To validate our model's specific assertion that CPSA is an abuse of role and power, we would expect to see evidence that pastors framed the experience of abuse as "being good for you" or otherwise consonant with pastoral guidance and counseling.

Perpetrators and Survivors: The Use of God to Leverage Sexual Exploitation

Farrell and Taylor's (2000) paper described how some CPSA perpetrators incorporate a distorted representation of a punitive, all-seeing God into their grooming of potential victims. According to this model, secrecy and silence are the core constructs that perpetuate the CPSA relationship. While secrecy and silence are not specific to this type of abuse, the strategy employed to obtain silence and secrecy may be different. Perpetrators may foster the feeling of being singled out for a special relationship with the perpetrator by God. In some cases, the feeling may be perpetuated by material rewards of gifts and special treatment by the perpetrator and/or the (promised) spiritual reward of "going to heaven." Additionally, clergymen could exploit the fear of being punished for denying both God's and the clergyman's will by distorting representations of what God "wants and needs." Anecdotally, clergymen have also twisted the confidentiality of pastoral counseling to maintain secrecy around CPSA. Furthermore, threats of excommunication, damnation, and other renderings of God's wrath have also been reported in the accounts of survivors. These strategies are similar to what is described with the traumagenic dynamic process of traumatic sexualization (Finkelhor & Browne, 1986) in which children are taught that rewards and punishments are contingent on their gratifying the perpetrator. Traumatic sexualization is strikingly evident in the case of one of Isely's (1996) respondents, a male survivor of CPSA who, reflecting on his years-long victimization, concluded: "The solution to problems [in my relationship with the clergy perpetrator] was to have sex" (p. 314).

Many church practices and customs become incorporated into this comprehensive silencing strategy. For example, absolute respect for all church leaders and officials can be manipulated to prevent defiance, disclosure, and escape. Secrecy is also highlighted in Summit's CSAAS model, in which secrecy is predicated on the child internalizing the perpetrator's threat that bad outcomes will happen if outsiders learn about the sexually abusive relationship. The negative outcome can be infliction of physical violence or public shame on the child or his or her loved ones, withdrawal of the perpetrator's positive attention, breakdown in the integrity and security of the home or parish (e.g., "They'll arrest me, you'll be taken away from your family, and your mother will be devastated"), or a combination of these. The frequent end result is the survivor acting in the role of co-conspirator to conceal his or her own abuse (Berliner & Conte, 1990; Furniss, 1991; German, Habenicht, & Futcher, 1990). Psychiatric symptoms and dysregulated behavior arise from the survivor's inner struggle to hold and make sense of contradictory messages in silence (e.g., "God is good, yet God is letting me be hurt" or "My pastor is kind and good, yet he hurts me").

We cannot draw on the extant literature to examine the concept of use of God to leverage sexual exploitation because the concepts are specific to CPSA. Thus, it is important for research to develop measures that specifically tap these and other unique facets of CPSA. Among the important dimensions that one might assess are the theological, existential, and spiritual domains both of the abuse itself and as part of the subsequent recovery. Farrell and Taylor (2000) described these domains in considerable detail and offer a helpful blueprint for how they might be operationalized. For example, the theological domain addresses survivors' difficulty reconciling abuse with the church's teachings, the existential domain survivors' damaged sense of life having value and meaning, and the spiritual domain survivors' feelings of losing God as a source of comfort and strength. In addition, qualitative analyses can begin to uncover the factors that are most relevant to maintaining silence and secrecy.

Perpetrators and Survivors: Betrayal, Powerlessness, and Damaged Self-Concept

Several models (Finkelhor & Browne, 1986; Summit, 1983) describe the corrosive power of sexual abuse on children's sense of self-worth, ability to trust that adults will keep them safe, and growing sense of powerlessness. Perpetrators can initiate this corrosive process by normalizing abnormal, developmentally inappropriate, often frightening sexual relations between a perpetrator and survivor. Learning to trust is an important milestone of psychosocial development that can be corrupted by CPSA (Erickson, 1950). The quotes of CPSA survivors are illustrative: "I would say as a child, I learned not to trust adults" and "[CPSA] destroys everything about how [children] feel about adults and about what sex did . . . to them" (Bera, 1995; p. 88). When the process of learning how to trust is disrupted by violence perpetrated by a caregiver or trusted adult, problems in psychological growth are likely to emerge (Herman, 1992). Some authors note that providers can expect to see hostility and other forms of disrupted attachment (e.g., clinginess), as well as dysregulated behavior.

These same concepts are also present in adult victims of CPSA, who often begin to question their own judgments about people to place faith in and/or trust. Similarly, this difficulty with trust is common in cases of intimate partner violence, where women sometimes lose all confidence in their ability to determine who is trustworthy and/or an appropriate partner. This process has been detailed in various models, including McFall's (1982) Social Information Processing Model, and may have direct relevance for adult women who are survivors of CPSA.

Powerlessness, another traumagenic dynamic, comes from the abuse-instilled sense that, ". . . nothing about me was mine. Everything about me belonged to someone else" (Bera, 1995, p. 89). The desperate need for mastery over something in the face of complete violation drives some children toward revictimization, sexualized behavior, aggression, and running away (see Kendall-Tackett, Williams, & Finkelhor, 1993, for prevalence statistics for these behaviors). A recent structural equation modeling study provided empirical support for the powerlessness and stigmatization dynamics mediating the effects of child sexual abuse severity on psychological distress in adult women (Kallstrom-Fuqua, Weston, & Marshall, 2004).

Self Discrepancy Theory is similar to the construct of powerlessness in that it can help to explain some of the interactive dynamics in CPSA relationships (Higgins, 1987, 1989b). Higgins proposed that perceived discrepancies between one's actual and ideal self-concept (actual-ideal discrepancy) will lead to depressed affect, whereas discrepancies between one's actual self and externally imposed standards for how one ought to be (actual-ought discrepancy) would lead to agitated, socially anxious feelings. Self-Discrepancy Theory seems particularly applicable to CPSA for a number of reasons. First, the construct resonates with anecdotal observations that some individuals refer to themselves as "good" or "bad" depending on how much they perceive themselves to be adhering to religious practices. Second, Higgins (1989a) proposed that the development of self-concept and the capacity to perceive discrepancies between the actual, ideal, and ought selves is developmentally mediated, specifically by Piagetian stages of cognitive development. Within this context, a wide range of behaviors from CPSA survivors are explainable. For example, if victimized boys are socialized to be tough and never to be a victim (Bolton, Morris, & MacEachron, 1989), then the CPSA survivor should be especially likely to experience actual-ought discrepancies that will lead to agitation and the disruptive behaviors that tend to bring them into treatment. Conversely, it would be beneficial to know if the higher rates of internalizing disorders in female children following trauma correspond to higher rates of actual-ideal discrepancy (Kendall-Tackett et al., 1993).

Fortunately, for those interested in examining these elements of betrayal, powerlessness, and self-concept in the role of CPSA, there are several studies to use as a foundation. For example, replication of Kallstrom-Fuqua and colleague's (2004) study using a sample of CPSA survivors could help to determine if powerlessness and stigma are mediating factors in the relationship between CPSA and psychological distress, as they are with other types of abuse. Similarly, it would be possible to examine self-discrepancies in CPSA survivors using Strauman and Higgins' (1988) methodology in a sample of CPSA survivors. Thus, the process of documenting the importance of betrayal, powerlessness, and self-concepts in CPSA are ripe for examination.

Perpetrators and Survivors: Predatory Clergy

Predatory clergymen are a small but clinically significant subgroup of perpetrating clergy. This type of perpetrator may be different from other types of perpetrating clergy in a number of quantitatively measurable ways, but from our perspective they qualitatively stand apart due to their apparently ego-syntonic antisociality and their remorseless willingness to use physical threats and aggression to satisfy their sexual needs. Evidence for this separate category of perpetrator is suggested by the fact that Hall and Hirschman's (1991) Quadripartite Model of Sexual Aggression fits the profile of nearly one-third of the alleged perpetrating priests detailed in the *National Clergy Sex Abuse Report* (NCSAR; The John Jay College Research Team, 2004) remarkably well,[1] but we stress: only one-third. As reported in the NCSAR (p. 39), 12% of 1,400 priests had documented histories of civil or criminal offenses, nearly 8% had documented problems with hostility, with an additional 26.5% for other personality-related problems, and nearly 4% had documented problems with coercive sex or "other sexual behavior." The NCSAR additionally reported that 13% of perpetrating priests had documented histories of being disciplined for having sex with adult partners, which for unknown reasons has been differentiated from the "coercive sex" category. Without survivor reports, we have no way to determine how much of this 13% is accounted for by truly "consensual" sexual relationships and how much may be best described as sexual misconduct as we described earlier. Given the power imbalance between clergy and parishioners, we must view with suspicion the possibility of any of these relationships being consensual.

One potential risk factor of sexually abusive behavior is the perpetrator's own history of being sexually abused. Meta-analyses reveal that 66% ($\eta^2 = .43$) of sexual abuse survivors showed developmentally inappropriate sexualized behavior, but not necessarily behavior that was sexually aggressive (Kendall-Tackett et al., 1993). The NCSAR found that a minority of accused priests (7%) endorsed a history of being abused themselves ($n = 274$). Of these 274 priests, the majority (65%) reported that they were sexually abused, and a smaller group (7%) endorsed being both sexually and physically abused. These data suggest that there may be a minority of individuals for whom violence and sexuality are inextricably linked. Unfortunately, this is true for a small subset of individuals in all walks of life. In cases where these individuals enter the ministry or other professions where they have authority over others, the results can be destructive to individuals with lesser authority.

In order to test this element of the model, specifically that predatory clergy are a unique subset of perpetrators, an assessment of motivational precursors to the abuse must be assessed. For example, it would ideally be possible to determine if clergymen experience sexual arousal to images of violence or degradation of women and/or children using empirical techniques such as the Barlow Strain Gauge (Barlow, Becker, Leitenberg, & Agras, 1970). Although certainly not a perfectly reliable method of testing, in combination with personality tests for sociopathy, emotion regulation difficulties (e.g., outbursts of anger), and careful clinical interviewing, it may be possible to document this profile.

Understanding the relationship between the perpetrator and survivor is critical to the understanding any type of abuse. We have outlined four mechanisms that can assist us in our understanding of this theme in CPSA. The abuse of power is inherently present in all cases of sexual abuse committed by clergy. This power dynamic is often complicated by the introduction of God, either overtly or covertly, into the abuse situation due to the clergyman's position in the community. These particular themes found in CPSA can profoundly impact a survivor's self-concept. Finally, the influence of predatory clergymen, although a minority of offenders, cannot be overestimated due to the callous and repeated incidences of their behavior.

THEME 2: RELATIONSHIPS BETWEEN SURVIVORS AND COMMUNITIES

The second theme examines the relationship between the survivor and the community in CPSA. Many authors describe how the experience of sexual violation in CPSA is compounded by rumor, scandal, and the withdrawal of social support within religious communities once the trauma is disclosed (Cooper-White, 1991; Fortune, 1989; Francis & Turner, 1995; Rediger, 1990). The result is an increasing sense of isolation from what used to be a safe haven. We postulate three factors that may contribute to the development and perpetuation of distress and impaired functioning for survivors, including the impact of others' disbelief, the role of shame, and community exclusion.

Survivors and Communities: The Impact of Others' Disbelief

According to Summit (1983), delayed, unconvincing disclosure is conceptualized as the behavioral consequence of three interactive processes.

First, the survivor may have been socialized to keep the abusive relationship secret to avoid catastrophe (as described earlier). Second, the survivor may feel helpless to change the situation. Third, perhaps to feel less helpless, the survivor may have convinced himself or herself that he or she can modulate the abuser's behavior by "being good." Under these conditions, the survivor will be unlikely to disclose, much less in a way that is convincing to fellow parishioners. Understandably, parishioners may collude with the survivor's unconvincing disclosure because they do not want to believe that such disturbing things can happen in "nice neighborhoods," parishes, or congregations.

Summit (1983) further conceptualizes survivor retraction as the behavioral manifestation of ambivalence: wanting to escape but feeling responsible for the welfare of loved ones. In the survivor's mind, this sense of responsibility is predicated on imagining that they need to keep the abuse secret in order to spare their loved ones from scandal and pain. A recent retrospective study of CSA survivors did not support the assertion that children make unconvincing disclosures or retract them, although it is important to note that delayed disclosure appeared to be normative (London, Bruck, Ceci, & Shuman, 2005). Nonetheless, Isely and Isely (1990) strongly recommended that those who might provide services for a child survivor of CPSA explore Summit's model and its utility for conceptualizing survivors' behavior.

Disclosing sexual abuse should ideally be considered a "cry for help" that leads to rescue of the survivor and corrective action toward the perpetrator. Disclosure is a vulnerable time for the survivor, and the response of their religious communities can alter or exacerbate their sense of worldview dissonance. A number of authors have described the strongly patriarchal culture of organized Christianity (Fishburn, 1982; Franz, 2002; Lothstein, 2002; Thoburn & Whitman, 2004) and used this to explain how it could create an atmosphere in which the presumed moral authority of the priest or minister is used to override the allegations and concerns of relatively disempowered groups, namely women and children. Children in particular are vulnerable to having their sense of right and wrong dictated by powerful adults. However, for survivors of all ages, disquieting dissonance is created when the clergyman, who defines morality for oneself, one's parents, and one's community, is also a perpetrator. We know that sexual abuse affects not only the survivor but also the people close to the survivor. The survivors' significant others may struggle to understand the changes in their loved one as a result of the abuse and to reconcile their feelings toward the perpetrator. Feelings of shock, confusion, and divided loyalty are common reactions in families in which incest has occurred (Courtois, 1988), and to the extent that religious communities have features in common with families, these reactions may also be applicable to CPSA. Fortune (1989) poignantly described six women's reports of feeling betrayed and ostracized by their church after they disclosed that their pastor sexually abused them. The words of one woman interviewed by Fortune are particularly powerful:

> It does pain me . . . that a number of people that I have known for many years, have worked with, have considered to be my friends, have chosen to blame the women for "chasing after [our pastor]," or have lightly dismissed the whole issue with remarks like "boys will be boys," despite the overwhelming evidence that [our pastor] was asked to leave two (and possibly five) churches for similar incidents of sexual misconduct. *On the other hand, I understand [our pastor's] tremendous power of persuasion and intimidation—and probably we must share some of the guilt for letting this kind of situation persist for so long a time.* (p. 95, our emphasis)

In addition to this passage highlighting how community disbelief can manifest in cases of CPSA, it is notable that Fortune's respondent to some degree internalizes blame for her victimization.

From a research perspective, it is important to be able to document the importance of responses to disclosure in recovery from CPSA. Qualitative data such as that collected by Fortune provide an excellent example of how these important research questions can be addressed. While it seems logical that community reaction to disclosure would be an important facet of recovery, this has not been examined directly with quantitative data in CPSA survivors. Using the Summit (1983) model, the retrospective research conducted by London and colleagues (2005) and Courtois' (1988) incest research as a guide, it may be possible to apply methods used with survivors of other types of abuse to the CPSA population. Additionally, development of CPSA–specific measures may assist in this type of research endeavor in the future.

Survivors and Communities: The Role of Shame

Shame may be an important mediating emotion in the potentially adversarial interaction between survivors and their religious communities. Proneness to experiencing shame has been found to be an important predictor of a variety of mental health outcomes in survivors of sexual abuse, usually accounting for additional variance beyond abuse severity (Andrews, Brewin, Rose, & Kirk, 2000; Feiring, Taska, & Lewis, 2000; Kessler & Bieschke, 1999; Talbot, Talbot, & Tu, 2004). In these studies, shame is defined as the desire to hide, disappear, or die due to feeling defective, often as the result of failing to meet one's own or others' internalized standards (Tangney, 1995). It is highly likely that this construct would be applicable to CPSA, given that churches are such powerful definers and enforcers of moral behavior. Shame is believed to be a fundamental motivator of "proper behavior," as when children are told that "God is watching" what they do, say, and think. The implicit assumption is that shame is so aversive to the person experiencing it that he or she will inhibit behaviors that would bring others' disapproval in the future.

However, one study suggests that high shame proneness may actually be a predictor of increased "wrongdoing." In a longitudinal study, fifth graders who were highly shame prone (measured by forced-choice responses to descriptions of moral dilemmas) had a significantly higher frequency of drug use and suspensions at age 18–19 than their less shame prone peers (Tangney & Dearing, 2002). Should this finding be replicated, it would suggest that highly shame prone survivors, and perhaps perpetrators, of CPSA would be especially likely to be trapped in an escalating negative spiral of abuse and destructive behavior. Shame may therefore be especially destructive in religious communities, where the survivor is made to feel simultaneously deserving of the abuse by the perpetrator and ostracized by the congregation for "falsely" accusing a beloved pastor. We explore the possible self-preserving motivations for ostracizing a survivor in the community exclusion section below.

In terms of empirical support, a next logical step in applying the research on shame to the CPSA population would be to replicate studies documenting the importance of this construct. Thus, it may be possible to document the importance of shame in terms of revictimization or maladaptive coping behaviors (e.g., substance abuse) in survivors of CPSA. Similarly, it would be important to determine if mental health outcomes are impacted by the presence of shame using similar methods to studies with other survivor populations (Andrews et al., 2000; Feiring et al., 2000; Kessler & Bieschke, 1999; Talbot et al., 2004).

Survivors and Communities: Community Exclusion

Rather than receiving acceptance and support from their communities, survivors of CPSA often report being excluded or ostracized by members of their community (see Neustein & Lesher, 2008). One rather severe example of exclusion in religious communities is "disfellowshipping" among Jehovah's Witnesses, in which an entire congregation, including blood relatives, will shun a congregant for various sins, including divorce, adultery, and "provocative dancing" (e.g., see silentlambs.org, n.d.). Terror Management Theory (TMT; Pyszczynski, Greenberg, & Solomon, 1997) may help explain this rejecting response by communities. TMT proposes that the fear of death, or "mortality salience," drives many social phenomena related to the preservation of self- and worldview. To simplify, no one likes to consider their own mortality. As such, people comfort themselves by creating a sense of safety through their social routines and beliefs. During times of physical or psychological threat, an individual's need for this sense of security increases, leading them to hold more steadfastly to their beliefs. In fact, when people are primed to think about their own mortality (using death-related words embedded in experimental tasks) they tend to reward people who agree with their worldview and punish those who do not. In other words, people tend to "derogate and punish those who violate cultural standards" as a method of reacting to their own mortality (Leary & Schreindorfer, 1997, p. 27; see also McGregor et al., 1998). TMT is a potential mediator in the relationship between a survivor disclosing abuse and the often victim-blaming, ostracizing stance taken by the religious community toward the survivor (e.g., Fortune, 1989; Francis & Turner, 1995; Isely, 1996). A number of TMT–informed studies have connected mortality salience to constructs that we believe are highly relevant to CPSA, such as attitudes toward sexuality (Goldenberg, Pyszczynski, McCoy, Greenberg, & Solomon, 1999), sex as a moral transgression (Rosenblatt, Greenberg, Solomon, Pyszczynski, & Lyon, 1989), group membership (Greenberg et al., 1990), and individuals who violate or criticize group norms (Dechesne, Janssen, & van Knippenberg, 2000). Further suggestive evidence that TMT would be applicable to CPSA is that the relationship between mortality salience and condemnation of moral transgressions appears to be generalizable across intrapersonal and interpersonal crimes (Florian & Mikulincer, 1997). In other words, mortality salience not only impels direct attacks on an individual for suspected moral transgressions, but also secondary harm to the wounded party's significant others and community.

To the extent that a survivor who discloses CPSA is seen as a critic of or threat to the religious community, derogation and condemnation is a very understandable outcome within the TMT framework. It is certainly easier to condemn a single "deviant"/outgroup member than to question the goodness of the clergyman who represents the entire religious community. This may be especially true for highly cloistered communities, such as the Amish, in which the church handles nearly all disputes and legal matters, including serious crimes (Pinto, 2004).

There are several studies of the central elements of TMT utilizing basic experimental paradigms. However, these constructs have not yet been examined directly in CPSA survivors and the community exclusion experienced by many of these survivors. A next important step would then be to test the effects of priming mortality awareness on behaviors and attitudes with both survivors and communities that have been impacted by CPSA. Clearly an important variable to assess in this type of experimentation would be the perceived permeability of group boundaries in religious communities.

Considering the central role the clergyman plays in the religious community and the importance of the community as a support for survivors, understanding the relationship between the survivor and the community is particularly important in CPSA. We have outlined three mechanisms that can assist in understanding this theme in CPSA. The impact of community disbelief when survivors recount their abuse is repeatedly noted and often closely linked to the experience of survivors' shame. In many cases, particularly in closed religious communities, survivors are deliberately excluded or shunned from institutions that were previously of central importance in their lives.

THEME 3: RELATIONSHIP BETWEEN CLERGYPERSON AND COMMUNITY

The third theme examines the relationship between clergyman and the community. In some respects, this is both the most ambitious and most tentative theme presented. Most authors who examine CPSA examine only limited aspects of the phenomenon and generally do not discuss perpetrators and survivors in the same paper. However, this is an initial attempt to provide an interactive dynamic model that accounts for the multiple layers that contribute to CPSA. Three themes are detailed: community ambivalence toward the perpetrator, cognitive style, and cognitive adaptability.

Clergymen and Community: Ambivalence Toward the Perpetrator

The literature about religious communities' reactions to disclosed abuse suggests that ambivalence toward perpetrating clergymen is common.

As in other forms of sexual abuse, reactions to disclosure seem to vary. One extreme response is a denial of the allegations coupled with a desire to protect the accused priest (e.g., Richards, 2004). The opposite extreme response includes a strong punitive demand for "zero tolerance," whereas a more moderate response can include a hopeful plea for rehabilitation (see e.g., McConnaha, 2002). An area of study that has direct relevance to this area is the literature concerning sexual misconduct perpetrated by an "impaired professional" (e.g., Layman & McNamara, 1997). Schoener and Gonsiorek (1988) identified six types of impaired psychotherapists who engage in sexual misconduct, ranging from the highly treatable and help-seeking "mildly neurotic" type to severely character-disordered types who lack remorse and are unlikely to benefit from treatment. Francis and Turner (1995) applied a very similar typology to clergy engaging in sexual misconduct, distinguishing between temporarily impaired, naïve, and "educable" clergymen and "those who have a world view that says they are entitled to have their needs met at the expense of others and may have to leave the clergy because of personality disorders" (p. 218). The degree to which sexual misconduct by clergy is pathologized or viewed as a training issue may vary even within the same denomination. For example, in one northeastern Episcopal diocese, seminarians in their final stages of training before ordination are supervised and evaluated on their progress in developing good pastoral boundaries, where failure to develop these boundaries may be grounds for termination from training (anonymous Episcopal postulant "A," personal communication, July 25, 2005). At the same time, it is not uncommon for Episcopal seminarians to hear their instructors speculate that sexual misconduct is a remediable condition arising from being overworked and overstressed (anonymous Episcopal postulant "B," personal communication, July 14, 2005).

Community ambivalence toward a clergyperson who has been accused of CPSA is a difficult construct to examine. This construct is difficult to examine in part due to the range of responses that might be present within one faith community. Each individual within the community may have a different reaction, whereas the community response is typically either an average of these responses or is characterized by a few vocal community members who may or may not represent the majority in the community. However, careful qualitative assessment may be the key to documenting a phenomenon that is often discussed anecdotally as being an important variable in communities that are coping with this type of accusation. Toward this end, we recommend the use of Grounded Theory, a rigorous method of extracting and testing constructs found in qualitative data (e.g., Strauss & Corbin, 1990). Only through thorough examination of the dynamic processes that occur between clergymen and their communities of faith can we begin to understand the ways in which these communities can begin to heal. In addition, by understanding underlying motives for perpetration and factors that allow CPSA to occur can we develop effective training and preventative programs.

Clergymen and Community: Cognitive Style

It is important when trying to understand the interactions of perpetrating clergymen with victims and the larger community that we consider the internal motivations and rationalizations for inappropriate behavior. For example, the Thought–Action–Fusion theoretical model (Steketee & Barlow, 2002) is one model that can help us understand a perpetrator's cognitive style. This model refers to the irrational belief that having a thought or urge is equivalent to performing the behavior and/or that thoughts increase the likelihood of a behavior's occurrence. Interestingly, there is a body of research that demonstrates that high levels of thought-action-fusion are present in individuals who identify themselves as highly religious (Rassin & Koster, 2003). In essence, this correlation suggests that highly religious individuals are more likely to believe that having a "sinful" thought is equivalent to perpetrating a "sinful" action or behavior.

Thought-action-fusion could be an important mediating variable in CPSA on several levels. Initially, it may be a factor in the clergyman's decision making to perpetrate. For example, they might believe themselves "damned" for having thoughts about perpetrating. Therefore, there would be no additional consequence for acting on these thoughts given that they believe that having the thoughts and urges are equivalent to acting on these feelings. Similarly, the congregation may reject a clergyman who is seeking assistance to resist thoughts or urges based on the belief that having thoughts are equivalent to actions. We hypothesize that thought-action-fusion is encouraged in some faiths and internalized by some clergymen, survivors, and congregants. Awareness of this tendency toward thought-action-fusion coupled with honest communication between communities and clergymen could potentially provide a method of primary prevention of CPSA in the future and warrants further study.

There would be several ways to document if cognitive style is an important facet of the relationship of the clergyman to the community.

Further exploration of the "actual-ought" discrepancy as it relates to the perpetrator's behavior would be important. Additionally, several possible studies could help to elucidate the role of thought-action-fusion as a possible precursor for abuse as well as a moderator of recovery.

Clergymen and Community: Cognitive Adaptability

Excluding the small proportion of sociopathic clergymen discussed earlier, the clinical literature suggests that perpetrating clergymen are conflicted about their behavior and motivations (e.g., Fones, Levine, Althof, & Risen, 1999). Indeed, they may be experiencing actual-ought discrepancy as described by Higgins (1987, 1989b) and discussed earlier in our section on "Perpetrators and Survivors: Betrayal, Powerlessness, and Damaged Self-Concept." Considering this, it would not be surprising that accused clergymen (and their congregations) would *want to believe* that they can gain control over their sexually compulsive behavior and resume their clerical duties, whether or not they actually can.[2]

TMT may also provide a means of understanding the cognitive adaptations made by perpetrating clergy on being discovered and accused. TMT suggests that an allegation of sexual misconduct is a powerful enough threat to one's symbolic life to activate the mechanisms of psychological self-preservation. In TMT, such a cognitive adaptation occurs largely outside of conscious awareness, but it would be as if the accused clergyman—and the devout parishioner—followed this line of thought:

> Clergy who sexually abuse parishioners are monsters and deserve punishment. For a clergyman, these punishments—excommunication, being "defrocked," etc.—are the functional equivalent of being killed, and this terrifies me. In order to survive as a clergyman/parishioner, I/ my clergyman must be capable of changing, and I/my clergyman have done enough good in my/his life that I believe that I am/my clergyman is different from those "other" sexually abusive clergy. My/my clergyman's case is different.

One way to test if such a cognitive adaptation occurs is to see whether measures of belief in one's rehabilitation positively correlate with other measures of rehabilitation. We must note here that we are not judging the veracity of perpetrating clergy's assertions that they can be helped but rather suggesting a psychological mechanism that could impel such assertions (and parishioners' desire to believe them), as well as a possible method to test this element of our theoretical model.

DISCUSSION

We have proposed a dynamic interactive model of CPSA that primarily focuses on the relationships between survivors, perpetrators, and their religious communities. We acknowledge that this interactive dynamic model is a complex one that would require extensive research to determine if the assertions are supported. However, we believe that this model can provide a foundation for future investigations. This model integrates the relatively small literature on CPSA with some of the more extensive literature on sexual trauma perpetrated by nonclergy. By using this broader framework as a base, we have attempted to provide an empirically testable model that also includes examples of supporting evidence where possible. While the possible research suggested throughout this manuscript is not meant to be exhaustive, we are hopeful that it will spur continued interest in this highly important phenomenon. Overall, we would argue for the continued need for qualitative research that has dominated the field of CPSA research to date. This research has predominately focused on the statements of survivors, thus we would argue for more in-depth qualitative research on the perpetrators and communities affected by CPSA. In this way, we can begin to examine this interactive set of dynamics.

In addition to qualitative studies, quantitative study is needed in this field. Fortunately, there are several related trauma-focused studies that can inform this literature. Wherever possible, drawing on the experience and knowledge of the extant literature would be important. For example, replicating some of the studies mentioned throughout this manuscript with populations of CPSA survivors, perpetrators, and communities would be important first steps for this literature. However, we also recognize that there is a need for specialized measurement tools for fully understanding this phenomenon. Therefore, we would encourage the development and validation of specialized assessment tools that tap some of the unique spiritual and philosophical domains of CPSA. Indeed, the problem of CPSA is a complex one that is not easily understood or solved. Nonetheless, we are hopeful that this comprehensive volume and the empirical and clinical work that might be stimulated from it will be rigorous and well-informed.

NOTES

1. Hall and Hirschman (1991) propose that four "motivational precursors" (p. 662) increase the likelihood of sexual aggression: physiological sexual arousal (sometimes associated with extremely inappropriate stimuli, such as children or violence); justifying cognitions (e.g., "women want or deserve to be raped"); affective dyscontrol (e.g., anger and hostility); and personality problems, particularly antisociality.

2. There is a literature on the rehabilitation of sexual offenders that is beyond the scope of this paper. Readers are referred to the work of McGrath (1991) and Hanson and Bussière (1998).

REFERENCES

Allers, C. T., Benjack, K. J., & Allers, N. T. (1992). Unresolved childhood sexual abuse: Are older adults affected? *Journal of Counseling & Development, 71*(1), 14–17.

Andrews, B., Brewin, C. R., Rose, S., & Kirk, M. (2000). Predicting PTSD symptoms in victims of violent crime: The role of shame, anger, and childhood abuse. *Journal of Abnormal Psychology, 109*(1), 69–73.

Associated Press. (2005, June 10–12). Church abuse scandal: $1 billion and counting. *Metro Boston Edition*, p. 1.

Barlow, D. H., Becker, R., Leitenberg, H., & Agras, W. (1970). A mechanical strain gauge for recording penile circumference change. *Journal of Applied Behavior Analysis, 6*, 355–367.

Bera, W. H. (1995). *Clergy sexual abuse and male survivors: A study of stress and coping among 25 men abused by the same minister during their adolescence.* Unpublished doctoral dissertation, University of Minnesota, Minneapolis, MN.

Berliner, L., & Conte, J. R. (1990). The process of victimization: The victims' perspective. *Child Abuse and Neglect, 14*(1), 29–40.

Bolton, F. G., Jr., Morris, L. A., & MacEachron, A. E. (1989). *Males at risk: The other side of child sexual abuse.* Newbury Park, CA: Sage Publications.

Cooper-White, P. (1991, February 20). Soul stealing: Power relations in pastoral sexual abuse. *Christian Century*, 196–199.

Courtois, C. A. (1988). *Healing the incest wound: Adult survivors in therapy.* New York: W. W. Norton & Company.

Dechesne, M., Janssen, J., & van Knippenberg, A. (2000). Derogation and distancing as terror management strategies: The moderating rule of need for closure and per-meability of group boundaries. *Journal of Personality and Social Psychology, 79*, 923–932.

Disch, E., & Avery, N. (2001). Sex in the consulting room, the examining room, and the sacristy: Survivors of sexual abuse by professionals. *American Journal of Orthopsy-chiatry, 71*(2), 204–217.

The Episcopal Church. (1979, September). Letter of institution of a minister. In *The Book of Common Prayer* (p. 557). New York: The Church Hymnal Corporation.

Erikson, E. H. (1950, 1985). *Childhood and society* (35th anniversary ed.). New York: Wiley.

Farrell, D. P., & Taylor, M. (2000). Silenced by God: An examination of unique character-istics within sexual abuse by clergy. *Counselling Psychology Review, 15*(1), 22–31.

Feiring, C., Taska, L., & Lewis, M. (2002). Adjustment following sexual abuse discovery: The role of shame and attributional style. *Developmental Psychology, 38*, 79–82.

Finkelhor, D., & Browne, A. (1986). Initial and long-term effects: A conceptual frame-work. In D. Finkelhor (Ed.), *A sourcebook on child sexual abuse* (pp. 180–198). Beverly Hills, CA: Sage Publications.

Fishburn, J. (1982). Male clergy adultery as vocational confusion. *Christian Century*, 922.

Florian, V., & Mikulincer, M. (1997). Fear of death and the judgment of social transgres-sions: A multidimensional test of terror management theory. *Journal of Personality and Social Psychology, 73*(2), 369–380.

Flynn, K. A. (2000). *Clergy sexual abuse of women: A specialized form of trauma.* Unpublished doctoral dissertation, Claremont Graduate University, Claremont, California.

Flynn, K. A. (2008). In their own voices: Women who were sexually abused by members of the clergy. *Journal of Child Sexual Abuse, 17*(3–4), 216–237.

Fones, C. L., Levine, S. B., Althof, S. E., & Risen, C. B. (1999). The sexual struggles of 23 clergymen: A follow-up study. *Journal of Sex and Marital Therapy, 25*, 183–195.

Fortune, M. (1989). *Is nothing sacred? When sex invades the pastoral relationship.* San Francisco: Harper & Row.

Francis, P. C., & Turner, N. R. (1995). Sexual misconduct within the Christian Church: Who are the perpetrators and those they victimize? *Counseling and Values, 39*, 218–227.

Franz, T. (2002). Power, patriarchy, and sexual abuse in the Christian church. *Traumatology, 8*, 1–12.

Frawley O'Dea, M. G., & Goldner, V. (Eds.). (2004). The sexual abuse crisis in the Catholic Church [Special issue]. *Gender & Sexuality, 5*(1–2).

Furniss, T. (1991). *The multi-professional handbook of child sexual abuse: Integrated management, therapy, and legal intervention.* London: Routledge.

Gagnon, M., & Hersen, M. (2000). Unresolved childhood sexual abuse and older adults: Late-life vulnerabilities. *Journal of Clinical Geropsychology, 6*(3), 187–198.

German, D. N., Habenicht, D. J., & Futcher, W. G. (1990). Psychological profile of the female adolescent incest victim. *Child Abuse and Neglect, 14*(3), 429–438.

Glaser, R. D., & Thorpe, J. S. (1986). Unethical intimacy: A survey of sexual contact and advances between psychology educators and female graduate students. *American Psychologist, 41*(1), 43–51.

Goldenberg, J. L., Pyszczynski, T., McCoy, S. K., Greenberg, J., & Solomon, S. (1999). Death, sex, love, and neuroticism: Why is sex such a problem? *Journal of Personality and Social Psychology, 77*(6), 1173–1187.

Goldner, V. (2004). The sexual abuse crisis and the Catholic Church: Gender, sexuality, power, and discourse. *Studies in Gender and Sexuality, 5*, 1–9.

Goodwin, J., Cormier, L., & Owen, J. (1983). Grandfather-granddaughter incest: A trigen-erational view. *Child Abuse and Neglect, 7*, 163–170.

Greenberg, J., Pyszczynski, T., Solomon, S., Rosenblatt, A., Veeder, M., Kirkland, S., et al. (1990). Evidence for terror management theory II: The effects of mortality salience on reactions to those who threaten or bolster the cultural worldview. *Journal of Personality and Social Psychology, 58*, 308–318.

Hall, G. C., & Hirschman, R. (1991). Toward a theory of sexual aggression: A quadripartite model. *Journal of Consulting and Clinical Psychology, 59*(5), 662–669.

Hanson, R. K., & Bussière, M. T. (1998). Predicting relapse: A meta-analysis of sexual offender recidivism studies. *Journal of Consulting and Clinical Psychology, 66*(2), 348–362.

Herman, J. (1992). *Trauma and recovery: The aftermath of violence—From domestic abuse to political terror.* New York: Basic Books.

Herman, J. (1993). Father-daughter incest. In J. P. Wilson & B. Raphael (Eds.), *International handbook of traumatic stress syndromes* (pp. 593–600). New York: Plenum.

Herman, J., & Hirschman, L. (1977). Father-daughter incest. *Signs: Journal of Women in Culture and Society, 2*(4), 735–756.

Herman, J., & Hirschman, L. (1981). Families at risk for father-daughter incest. *American Journal of Psychiatry, 138*(7), 967–970.

Higgins, E. T. (1987). Self-discrepancy: A theory relating self and affect. *Psychological Review, 94*, 319–340.

Higgins, E. T. (1989a). Continuities and discontinuities in self-regulatory and self-evaluative processes: A developmental theory relating self and affect. *Journal of Personality, 57*(2), 407–444.

Higgins, E. T. (1989b). Self-discrepancy theory: What patterns of self-beliefs cause people to suffer? *Advances in Experimental Social Psychology, 22*, 93–136.

Hunter, M. (1990). *Abused boys: The neglected victims of sexual abuse.* New York: Fawcett Books.

Isely, P. J. (1996). *In their own voices: A qualitative study of men sexually abused as children by Catholic clergy.* Unpublished doctoral dissertation, Boston University School of Education, Boston, Massachusetts.

Isely, P. J., & Isely, P. (1990). The sexual abuse of male children by church personnel: Intervention and prevention. *Pastoral Psychology, 39*(2), 85–99.

Isely, P. J., Isley, P., Freiburger, J., & McMackin, R. (2008). In their own voices: A qualitative study of men abused as children by Catholic clergy. *Journal of Child Sexual Abuse 17*(3–4), 201–215.

Jewish sexual abuse. (n.d.). Retrieved June 5, 2005, from http://www.the7thfire.com/new_world_order/zionism/jewish_sexual_abuse.html.

The John Jay College Research Team. (2004, February 27). *The nature and scope of the problem of sexual abuse of minors by Catholic priests and deacons in the United States: A research study conducted by the John Jay College of Criminal Justice (National Clergy Sex Abuse Report).* Retrieved April 13, 2005, from http://www.jjay.cuny.edu/churchstudy/main.asp.

Kallstrom-Fuqua, A. C., Weston, R., & Marshall, L. L. (2004). Childhood and adolescent sexual abuse of community women: Mediated effects on psychological distress and social relationships. *Journal of Consulting and Clinical Psychology, 72*(6), 980–992.

Kendall-Tackett, K. A., Williams, L. M., & Finkelhor, D. (1993). Impact of sexual abuse on children: A review and synthesis of recent empirical studies. *Psychological Bulletin, 113*(1), 164–180.

Kessler, B. L., & Bieschke, K. J. (1999). A retrospective analysis of shame, dissociation, and adult victimization in survivors of childhood sexual abuse. *Journal of Consulting and Clinical Psychology, 46*, 335–341.

Kohlenberg, R. J., & Tsai, M. (1998). *Healing interpersonal trauma with the intimacy of the therapeutic relationship.* New York: Guilford Press.

Layman, M. J., & McNamara, J. R. (1997). Remediation for ethics violations: Focus on psychotherapists' sexual contact with clients. *Professional Psychology: Research and Practice, 28*(3), 281–292.

Leary, M. R., & Schreindorfer, L. S. (1997). Unresolved issues with terror management theory. *Psychological Inquiry, 8*, 26–29.

London, K., Bruck, M., Ceci, S. J., & Shuman, D. W. (2005). Disclosure of child sexual abuse: What does the research tell us about the ways that children tell? *Psychology, Public Policy, and Law, 11*, 194–226.

Lothstein, L. M. (2002). Treating clergy who sexually abuse minors: A 16-year experience in the Professionals and Clergy Program at the IOL. *Connecticut Psychologist, 56*, 1, 4.

McConnaha, S. (2002, May 2). Priests called together to discuss clergy abuse issue. Series of upcoming listening sessions, a result of gathering. *The Milwaukee Catholic Herald.* Retrieved July 6, 2005, from http://www.chnonline.org/2002/2002-05-02/index.html.

McFall, R. M. (1982). A review and reformulation of the concept of social skills. *Behavioral Assessment, 4*, 1–33.

McGlone, G. J. (2003). The pedophile and the pious: Towards a new understanding of sexually offending and non-offending Roman Catholic priests. *Journal of Aggression, Maltreatment and Trauma, 8*(1-2), 115–131.

McGrath, R. J. (1991). Sex offender risk assessment and disposition planning: A review of the empirical and clinical findings. *International Journal of Offender Therapy and Comparative Criminology, 35*(4), 328–349.

McGregor, H. A., Greenberg, J., Arndt, J., Lieberman, J. D., Solomon, S., Simon, L., et al. (1998). Terror management and aggression: Evidence that mortality salience motivates aggression against worldview-threatening others. *Journal of Personality and Social Psychology, 74*, 590–605.

McLaughlin, B. R. (1994). Devastated spirituality: The impact of clergy sexual abuse on the survivor's relationship with God and the church. *Sexual Addiction & Compulsivity, 1*, 145–158.

Neustein, A., & Lesher, M. (2008). A single-case study of rabbinic sexual abuse in the orthodox Jewish community. *Journal of Child Sexual Abuse, 17*(3–4), 270–289.

Paulson, M. (2005, April 3). Late in pontiff's reign, clergy sex abuse case rocked the church. *The Boston Globe Online.* Retrieved April 12, 2005, from http://www.boston.com/news.

Pearlin, L. J., & Schooler, C. (1987). The structure of coping. *Journal of Health and Social Behavior, 19*, 2–21.

Penfold, P. S. (1999). Why did you keep going for so long? Issues for survivors of long-term, sexually abusive "helping" relationships. *Journal of Sex Education and Therapy, 24*(4), 244–251.

Pinto, B. (2004, October 22). Sex abuse case shocks Amish community: Amish woman ends silence, reports brothers' sexual abuse. *ABC News Online*. Retrieved July 14, 2005, from http://abcnews.go.com/WNT/story?id=189191&page=1.

Pyszczynski, T., Greenberg, J., & Solomon, S. (1997). Why do we need what we need? A terror management perspective on the roots of human social motivation. *Psychological Inquiry, 8*, 1–20.

Rassin, E., & Koster, E. (2003). The correlation between thought-action fusion and religiosity in a normal sample. *Behavior Research and Therapy, 41*(3), 361–368.

Rediger, L. G. (1990). *Ministry and sexuality, cases, counseling, and care*. Minneapolis, MN: Fortress.

Resick, P. A., Schnicke, M. K., & Markway, B. G. (1991, November). *Personal beliefs and reactions scale: The relation between cognitive content and posttraumatic stress disorder*. Paper presented at the 25th annual convention of the Association of the Advancement of Behavior Therapy, New York, NY.

Richards, A. F. C. (2004). Sexual misconduct by clergy in the Episcopal Church. *Studies in Gender and Sexuality, 5*(2), 139–165.

Rosenblatt, A., Greenberg, J., Solomon, S., Pyszczynski, T., & Lyon, D. (1989). Evidence for terror management theory: I. The effects of mortality salience on reactions to those who violate and uphold cultural values. *Journal of Personality and Social Psychology, 57*, 681–690.

Rossetti, S. J. (1995). The impact of child sexual abuse on attitudes toward God and the Catholic Church. *Child Abuse and Neglect, 19*(12), 1469–1481.

Russell, D. E. (1986). *The secret trauma: Incest in the lives of girls and women*. New York: Basic Books.

Schoener, G. R., & Gonsiorek, J. (1988). Assessment and development of rehabilitation plans for counselors who have sexually exploited their clients. *Journal of Counseling and Development, 67*(4), 227–232.

Silentlambs.org. (n.d.). *Abused lambs speak out*. Retrieved July 14, 2005, from http://www.silentlambs.org/personal_experiences/abused_lambs.cfm.

Simpkinson, A. A. (1996, November/December). Soul betrayal: Sexual abuse by spiritual leaders violates trust, devastates lives, and tears communities apart. No denomination or tradition is immune [Electronic version]. *Common Boundary*. Retrieved June 22, 2005, from http://www.advocateweb.org/hope/soulbetrayal.asp.

Steketee, G., & Barlow, D. H. (2002). Obsessive-compulsive disorder. In D. H. Barlow (Ed.), *Anxiety and its disorders: The nature and treatment of anxiety and panic* (2nd ed., pp. 516–550). New York: Guilford Press.

Strauman, T. J., & Higgins, E. T. (1988). Self-discrepancies as predictors of vulnerability to distinct syndromes of chronic emotional distress. *Journal of Personality, 56*(4), 685–707.

Strauss, A., & Corbin, J. M. (1990). *Basics of qualitative research: Grounded theory procedures and techniques*. Thousand Oaks, CA: Sage Publications.

Summit, R. C. (1983). The child sexual abuse accommodation syndrome. *Child Abuse and Neglect, 7*(2), 177–193.

Talbot, J. A., Talbot, N. L., & Tu, X. (2004). Shame-proneness as a diathesis for dissociation in women with histories of childhood sexual abuse. *Journal of Traumatic Stress, 17*, 445–448.

Tangney, J. P. (1995). Recent advances in the empirical study of shame and guilt. *American Behavioral Scientist, 38*, 1132–1145.

Tangney, J. P., & Dearing, R. (2002). *Shame and guilt.* New York: Guilford Press.

Thoburn, J., & Whitman, M. (2004). Clergy affairs: Emotional investment, longevity of relationship and affair partners. *Pastoral Psychology, 52*(6), 491–506.

The Impact of Clergy-Perpetrated Sexual Abuse: The Role of Gender, Development, and Posttraumatic Stress

Jason M. Fogler
Jillian C. Shipherd
Stephanie Clarke
Jennifer Jensen
Erin Rowe

Clergy-perpetrated sexual abuse (CPSA) has received more attention in recent years due to increased media focus on the sequelae of these events for survivors of CPSA (see e.g., *Christian Ethics Today*, 2000). The National Clergy Sex Abuse Report (NCSAR; The John Jay College Research Team, 2004) indicated that 10,667 claims of CPSA were made between 1950 and 2002. Four thousand clerics were accused of sexual abuse over 50 years, which comprised 4% of all Catholic clerics in the United States. Between 1984 and 1994, more than 5,000 survivors in the United States confronted church officials about CPSA (Farrell & Taylor, 1999).

When considered with other forms of sexual abuse, CPSA is part of a widespread problem of nearly epidemic proportions. The NCSAR (The John Jay College Research Team, 2004) revealed the gravity and pervasiveness of sexual abuse as a problem, particularly for male children, while the World Health Organization (2001) exposed the global crisis of sexual violence against girls and women, citing very high rates of posttraumatic stress disorder (PTSD) and severe psychiatric illness in these populations.

Compared with the relatively small body of research on CPSA to date, the psychological sequelae and treatment of sexual abuse has been examined to a much greater degree in other survivor populations, such as children who have been sexually abused by nonclergy (Kendall-Tackett, Williams, & Finkelhor, 1993), adult survivors of incest (Chu, 1998; Herman, 1992), adult women raped by strangers or dating partners (Harned, 2004; Resick, Nishith, Weaver, Astin, & Feuer, 2002), and those abused by counselors or therapists (Bonosky, 1995; Disch & Avery, 2001; Pope, Levenson, & Schover, 1979; Pope, Schover, & Levenson, 1980; Underwood, 2002). The literature on recovery from sexual abuse, incest, and rape in children and adult women provides an important point of departure from which to consider the deleterious effects of CPSA. Research on other forms of sexual abuse and rape demonstrate that sequelae of these types of events can include mood disorders, substance abuse, behavioral dysregulation (including suicidality and self-injurious behavior), dissociation, anxiety, PTSD, and personality disorder (Chu). However, it is important to recognize that there are also unique factors associated with CPSA. In fact, a number of writers have considered the influence of patriarchal religious attitudes (Franz, 2002), clerical training and gender socialization in religious communities (Fishburn, 1982; Lothstein, 2002; Thoburn & Whitman, 2004), and the idea of survivors feeling "silenced by God" due to perpetrators' manipulation (Farrell & Taylor, 2000, p. 22). These unique religious-socialization factors may have direct relevance when considering the impact of CPSA. Thus, our goal is to synthesize what is currently known about the effects of other types of sexual abuse while also considering those effects that might be unique to CPSA.

Elsewhere in this volume (Fogler, Shipherd, Rowe, Jensen, & Clarke, 2008), we outlined a theoretical framework for understanding CPSA as the dynamic interaction between perpetrator, survivor, and religious community. This theoretically grounded approach to treatment may be beneficial to clinicians who are struggling with the daunting challenge of CPSA and its aftermath. At the same time, there may be additional nuances beyond the larger theoretical issues that need to be attended to in work with a survivor who is in an acute state of distress. We have therefore identified gender and development as potentially important client-specific factors in CPSA outcomes. As with our theoretical framework, we view theories of gender and development as lenses through which we can begin to understand (and hopefully intervene on) the microprocesses underlying the very complex and multifaceted problem of CPSA.

We highlight development and gender as potential moderators of CPSA outcome because quantitative and anecdotal evidence suggest that the two modal populations of CPSA survivors are latency-age and pre-to-early adolescent boys and adult women (e.g., Lothstein, 2002). The quantitative data strongly identify boys as an at-risk population for CPSA. According to the NCSAR, 81% of CPSA survivors are male, with boys between the ages of 11 and 14 constituting over 40% of all survivors. For comparison purposes, epidemiological estimates reveal much lower rates of sexual abuse in males within the general population (3% to 25%) as compared with females (10% to 64%) before the age of 18 (Salter, 1992). Evidence for adult women being a modal CPSA–survivor population come predominantly from small-sample qualitative studies (Flynn, 2000; Fortune, 1989) and from women being at higher risk for sexual assault in the general population (Norris, Foster, & Weisshaar, 2002).

The majority of this article will focus on hypothesized differences in the manifestation of CPSA–related symptomatology based on developmental stage and gender. In our view, the common ground for these survivor populations is the psychologically damaging and pathogenic effects of the perpetrating clergyman's abuse of role and power. Research suggests that CPSA is similar in its effects to sexual exploitation by medical and mental health professionals (Disch & Avery, 2001; Underwood, 2002) and clinical supervisors in the helping professions (Bonosky, 1995; Pope et al., 1979, 1980), with comparable expectations in terms of sequelae and treatment. Bonosky (1995) used the construct of *fiduciary responsibility* to define what lies at the core of these forms of abuse:

> a broad obligation to act in a client's "best interests" and refrain from exploitation and harm . . . fiduciary accountability can apply to any relationship that necessitates a "blind" trust of a professional's special knowledge or skills, such as those of an attorney, doctor, therapist, or educator. (p. 81)

We would unequivocally add priest, rabbi, pastor, and any other titles of religious leadership to Bonosky's list of professions. That said, CPSA is a highly sensitive topic that has direct relevance for the community of clergy, survivors and their families, and whole congregations. For this reason, we feel that it is important to state our stance on the topic of CPSA clearly and to provide a disclaimer about the limited scope of this paper.

DISCLAIMER

We unequivocally consider sexually abusive behavior to be dangerous and therefore requiring emergent intervention (see Isely & Isely, 1990 for an example of this position applied to the specific topic of CPSA). Other writers have thoughtfully suggested ways in which clergy leaders and congregations might handle the disclosure of CPSA and ways to provide a fair hearing, rehabilitation, and/or punishment to the alleged perpetrator (Fortune, 1989; Hardman-Cromwell, 1991). For these reasons, we will not be addressing the issue of clergy perpetrators or community interventions in this paper. The focus of this paper is on the impact of CPSA on survivors. Our expertise is in the applied and theoretical research, diagnosis, and treatment of PTSD in adult and child survivors (both male and female) of trauma. We will apply this expertise to the question of how the posttraumatic sequelae of CPSA may differ as a function of age and gender. Our goal is to stimulate hypothesis-driven work on a clinically important but relatively understudied topic. Without empirical support, we are far from being able to give any kind of "final word" on CPSA, but we are hopeful that our review of the literature will begin to address some of the unique barriers to disclosure and treatment-relevant issues that are specific to this population of survivors.

DEFINITIONS

In our review of the literature, we have followed the NCSAR's definition of "sexual abuse of a minor":

> sexual abuse includes contacts or interactions between a child and an adult when the child is being used as an object of sexual gratification for the adult. A child is abused whether or not this activity involves explicit force, whether or not it involves genital or physical contact, whether or not it is initiated by the child, and whether or not there is discernible harmful outcome. (The John Jay College Research Team, 2004, p. 12)

We chose this working definition because it is sufficiently broad to subsume both overtly sexual behavior (e.g., fondling, kissing, and oral, digital, or genital penetration) and less prototypical sexualized behaviors (e.g., exhibitionism, voyeurism, and exposure to sexually explicit material). This broad definition is consistent with the thinking of such writers as Harned (2004), who observed that a wide range of "unwanted sexual experiences" contributed equally to reported psychological distress in undergraduate women. In addition, we will go a step beyond the NCSAR and apply this definition to both child and adult survivors of CPSA in this paper. We will use the term "child sexual abuse" (CSA) to refer to the general category of sexual abuse of children, "clergy-perpetrated sexual abuse" (CPSA) to refer to sexual abuse perpetrated against any individual by members of the clergy, and, when necessary, we will use such clarifying terms as "CPSA of adult women and/or children" to discuss subgroups.

OVERVIEW

First, we will discuss the PTSD diagnosis, its application to sexual abuse generally, and its application to CPSA in particular. Second, we will discuss child development and gender as important moderating factors in the relationship between CPSA and its sequelae. Third, we will discuss what we know about treatment and recovery from other types of sexual abuse and extend this discussion to the clinical implications of gender and development for the initial presentation and treatment course of CPSA survivors. In this third section, we will also anticipate potential barriers to CPSA survivors disclosing that they have been abused, a necessary step to accessing treatment. Finally, we offer recommendations for future clinical research into the assessment, treatment, and potential moderating factors of recovery from CPSA.

TRAUMA AND PTSD

PTSD can occur following exposure to an event where a person's life or physical integrity was threatened and the individual felt fear, helplessness, or horror (American Psychiatric Association, 2000). Prototypically qualifying traumatic events for a diagnosis of PTSD include witnessing or directly suffering a physical or sexual assault, natural disaster, or war. The disorder is characterized by intrusive reexperiencing symptoms, avoidance of activities, thoughts and emotions associated with the event, and hyperarousal.

One of the hallmark symptoms of PTSD is upsetting thoughts and images that occur about the traumatic event, either through memories, nightmares, or dissociative flashbacks. This reexperiencing is accompanied by chronic hyperarousal, including exaggerated startle, anger, difficulty sleeping or concentrating, and hypervigilance for signs that the trauma may happen again. PTSD is also characterized by extreme avoidance of traumatic reminders (often through alcohol/substance abuse), emotional numbing, and/or isolating from friends and family (Keane & Barlow, 2002).

Individuals with PTSD describe themselves as fundamentally changed after experiencing trauma: formerly enjoyed pursuits and relationships seem less pleasurable, life seems shorter and bleaker, and the world seems far more dangerous (Herman, 1992). For some survivors of trauma, recovery will be challenged by additional traumatic events (Desai, Arias,

Thompson, & Basile, 2002; Kessler & Bieschke, 1999; Maker, Kemmelmeier, & Peterson, 2001; Marx, Heidt, & Gold, 2005), feelings of low self-esteem and worthlessness, dissociation from internal emotional states and external reality, chronic physical symptoms and somatization, interpersonal difficulties, and comorbid substance abuse (Chu, 1998; Shipherd, Stafford, & Tanner, 2005; Terr, 1991; Wagner & Linehan, 1998). This type of presentation is sometimes referred to as "complex PTSD." In addition to these severe psychiatric comorbidities, PTSD has also been found to have a negative impact on physical health (e.g., Schnurr & Jankowski, 1999). Health-related problems associated with PTSD include diabetes, cancer, thyroid disease, obesity, heart disease and hypertension, high cholesterol, liver disease, arthritis, and asthma and lung disease (e.g., Felitti, 1991; Golding, 1994; Rheingold, Acierno, & Resnick, 2004).

Reviews of the PTSD literature underscore that it is common for individuals to experience one or more traumatic events in their lifetime, but that only a fraction will go on to develop PTSD (Keane & Barlow, 2002; Keane, Weathers, & Foa, 2000; Resick & Calhoun, 2001). The most frequently cited statistics on this phenomenon come from the National Comorbidity Survey (NCS; Kessler, Sonnega, Bromet, Hughes, & Nelson, 1995), which found an overall trauma exposure rate of 60% for men and 51% for women, compared to a more modest overall PTSD prevalence rate of 7.8%. However, the NCS also found that certain types of trauma, rape in particular, are associated with higher rates of PTSD and that women appeared to experience higher rates of PTSD than men (10.4% versus 5.0%, respectively), perhaps due to the types of events they are likely to experience. Resick and Calhoun listed differential trauma types and rates of PTSD for men and women surveyed by the NCS. For men, the highest rates of PTSD were associated with reported experience of rape (65%), combat exposure (39%), childhood neglect (24%), and childhood physical abuse (22%). Women showed a similar pattern, with reported experiences of rape (46%) and childhood physical abuse (49%) showing the highest rates of PTSD, followed by threat with a weapon (33%),[1] sexual molestation (27%), and physical attack (21%). These statistics underscore the undeniable connection between sexual trauma and psychopathology, which has direct relevance to CPSA.

The literature strongly suggests that there are several factors that contribute to psychiatric symptoms and the likelihood of having a chronic course. These factors include sexual abuse that begins before age 16, abuse that goes undisclosed and untreated for extended periods of time,

abuse that is frequent and severe, abuse perpetrated by a parent or parental figure, and lack of social support in response to disclosure of the abuse
(Herman, Russell, & Trocki, 1986; Kendall-Tackett et al., 1993; Lovett,
2004; Maker et al., 2001; Mennen, 1993). Unfortunately, many of these
risk factors are present in boys who are survivors of CPSA, such as abuse
prior to age 16, abuse by a parental figure, and length of time to disclosure
(Bera, 1995; Celenza, 2004; Isely, 1996; Ponton & Goldstein, 2004;
Somer & Szwarcberg, 2001). Similarly, women who experience CPSA
often do not disclose the abuse for a long period of time, were abused by a
parental figure, often experience frequent and severe abuse, and seldom
find social support in response to the disclosure (Flynn, 2000).

RELEVANCE OF PTSD TO CPSA

Three doctoral dissertations noted the presence of PTSD–like symptomatology in adult survivors of CPSA. Two of these dissertations studied reactions to CPSA in male survivors who were abused as adolescents
(Bera, 1995; Isely, 1996), and the third studied women who were coerced
into sexual relationships with clergy as either children or young adults
(Flynn, 2000). Although the studies varied in methodology, each noted
problems in interpersonal relationships, affect regulation, and self-concept
following CPSA. Interestingly, these studies identified a common course
of response over the period of abuse: survivors initially felt special to
have been "singled out" by the charismatic clergy-perpetrator, but then
reported feeling conflicted and confused during the abuse and ultimately
feeling betrayed and alienated from their churches after the abuse had
ended. These studies allude to both the modal populations of CPSA survivors (boys between 11 and 14 and adult women) and to the importance of
examining the developmental factors and gender differences that could
influence course and treatment prognosis.

Farrell and Taylor (2000) considered the PTSD diagnosis to be a useful
starting point to begin understanding the sequelae of CPSA but concluded
that "there are qualitative differences in [CPSA-related] symptomatology,
which the PTSD diagnosis cannot explain" (p. 28). For example, the
CPSA–related symptoms cited by Farrell and Taylor include self-blame,
guilt, psychosexual disturbances, self-destructive behaviors (including
suicidality and parasuicidality), substance abuse, and revictimization.
This symptom profile is perhaps better captured by the "complex PTSD"
construct posited by Herman (1992) to explain the sequelae of chronic

sexual abuse or torture. Farrell and Taylor additionally commented, "[W]hat seems unique to survivors of [CPSA] are idiosyncratic trauma characteristics, which include theological, spiritual, and existential symptomatologies" (p. 28) (see Neustein & Lesher, 2008).

In sum, there are several potential pathways following CPSA. Some are marked by resilience, hardiness, and positive outcomes. Other pathways can include disruption in functioning in some circumscribed areas (e.g., avoidance of organized religions; McLaughlin, 1994), whereas others may follow a disastrous trajectory toward chronic posttraumatic symptomatology, inability to navigate interpersonal relationships, and avoidance of spiritual and personal growth (Herman, 1992; Ruzek, Polusny, & Abueg, 1998). We now consider two potentially important moderators of symptom severity in CPSA: development and gender.

DEVELOPMENT AS A MODERATING FACTOR IN CPSA

Across interpersonal, psychological, and neurobiological domains, trauma can have disastrous effects on child development (Cicchetti & Lynch, 1993; Duncan, 1996; Osofsky & Scheeringa, 1997). The transition from childhood to adolescence (ages 11–14) is the developmental period when CPSA occurred for many of the male children surveyed in the NCSAR. Graber and Brooks-Gunn (1996) posited that healthy development is facilitated by a "goodness of fit" between the developing child and an ideally sensitive and supportive environment at key transition points. What then happens when sexual abuse disrupts the normal dialectic between child and environment, especially when the religious community is supposed to represent the highest standard of sensitivity and supportiveness? To answer this question, we will discuss development in three domains that we feel are most relevant to and impacted by CPSA: physical maturation, cognitive maturation, and psychosocial developmental stage.

ROLE OF PHYSICAL MATURATION IN CPSA

The relatively young ages of male CPSA survivors may be partially explained by the fact that a perpetrator will (on average) have greater success in overpowering a prepubescent boy than a large adolescent male who is likely to have high levels of muscle-building, aggression-mediating testosterone (see Brooks-Gunn, 1991 for review). Beyond this reduction-ist formulation based on physical power alone, Bolton, Morris, and MacEachron (1989) considered the dynamics of family life and its impact on vulnerability to CPSA. In particular, they discussed the role of differ-ent types of parental attitudes toward male children's physical maturation and growing sexual curiosity. Ideally, the child's guardians will create a safe place where a boy can learn that the changes in his body and feelings are normal and what implications those changes have for safe sexual behavior in the future. Male children who experience CPSA can come from less cohesive homes and/or homes that entrust the child's education and care to trusted clergypersons (Bolton et al., 1989). It is notable that survivors are often enticed into abusive sexual activity with clergypersons after first being exposed to other taboo activities, such as drinking alco-hol, smoking cigarettes, or watching pornography (Isely & Isely, 1990). More research is needed to determine what links, if any, there are between the child's curiosity about sexual and other adult behaviors and these targeted grooming behaviors by abusive clergypersons.

ROLE OF COGNITIVE MATURATION IN CPSA

Piagetian theory suggests that children between the ages of 9 and 13, the modal age range of child CPSA survivors, are likely to be in either the third or fourth stages of cognitive sophistication or transitioning between the two (see Hetherington & Parke, 1993 for review). Key elements in the shift between the third Concrete Operational stage and the fourth Formal Operational stage at roughly age 11–12 are: (a) a shift from (concrete operational) deductive reasoning tied to observable phenomena to the (formal operational) capacity to formulate theories and test hypotheses using mental representation and abstract principles; (b) an increase in cog-nitive flexibility and abstraction; and (c) a shift from egocentric thinking to multiple perspective-taking. As the names imply, concrete operational reasoning is grounded in the physical world and the five senses, whereas formal operational reasoning is symbolic and imaginative. Broadly speak-ing, children in the concrete operational stage can be taught basic princi-ples of physical science (e.g., Newton's laws of motion, how light can be refracted through a prism), but until the child achieves formal operational reasoning, he or she will not be able to understand such theoretical concepts as using light-years to approximate the distance of stars or density to explain why a large piece of wood floats in water but a small piece of lead sinks. Far from being a homogeneous group, child survivors of CPSA will have considerable variability in their capacity to distinguish their own perspective from another's, to think flexibly and abstractly about what is happening to them, or to reconcile such conflicting information as a clergyperson being very kind in public but sexually abusive in private.

The implication of Piagetian theory for CPSA is that the modal age of abuse for boys occurs at a critical developmental period when they are forming an understanding of the world. What then happens when this understanding is formed in the context of overwhelming sexual activity with a trusted priest or pastor? When learning experiences are abusive or disrupted by the sequelae of abuse, the probability of forming distorted cognitions about oneself and the world is high. A child in the concrete operational stage, seeking straightforward answers for how the world works, may be particularly vulnerable to a trusted clergyperson's explanation that sex between adults and children is normal and that fear is a natural part of "trying something new." During this important transition to adolescence, children are just beginning to understand the idea that a stimulus can simultaneously produce both positive and negative emotional states (Harter & Buddin, 1987), and from this standpoint CPSA can be extremely harmful to a child's later ability to regulate emotions and impulses. On the other hand, a child in the formal operational stage may be able to see all too clearly how inappropriate the abusive relationship is, but his new capacity to imagine shaming one's parents or community as a consequence of breaking his silence opens a new door of vulnerability. In other words, if Piagetian theory holds true, then younger children would be more vulnerable to being "tricked" (e.g., "It was gross, but Fr. Joe said it was okay, because everyone does it, and I believed him") and older children would be more vulnerable to being "trapped" (e.g., "I knew it was wrong, but Fr. Joe said that the whole church could fall apart if people knew").

Regarding Farrell and Taylor's (2000) discussion of how perpetrators incorporate God into coercion of the child, children at different Piagetian stages will also have very different abilities to conceptualize God. Tied to the physical world, younger children in the concrete operational phase will be less able to separate the metaphysical God from God's human proxy (the abusive clergyperson), especially when the child is being told by the clergyperson what God needs, wants, and does to those who obey or defy Him. On the other hand, many of the existential, theological, and spiritual symptoms of CPSA described by Farrell and Taylor require the capacity for formal operational reasoning because of their symbolic and metaphysical foci. For example, a survivor may question God's benevolence (theological), feel robbed of his faith and identity as a religious person (existential), or experience "discomfort with religion assuming ownership of the spirit" (spiritual) (p. 29).[2] However, the role of these theoretical concepts need to be confirmed through research.

ROLE OF PSYCHOSOCIAL DEVELOPMENT IN CPSA

Erikson (1950/1985) wrote that throughout the lifespan, people must resolve eight core psychosocial conflicts ("Ages of Man"). These conflicts are psychosocial (i.e., psychologically and socially based) because they involve balancing individual needs with the demands of "society" broadly defined, be it parental discipline, company policy, or the nation's laws. Again, the ideal scenario is "goodness of fit" between the child and his or her environment with successful resolution of each stage leading to an increasing sense that one can fulfill most if not all of one's needs as long as one follows the appropriate rules and laws. The stages build on one another so that unsuccessful resolution of one phase can carry forward and affect development through later phases. Abuse and revictimization would be expected to negatively impact this process, creating neurotic fixations in all the phases when the abuse occurred. For example, Herman (1992) was particularly concerned with how issues of trust and mistrust were affected by abuse. For example, "How safe can the world be if my own priest raped me, and my parents want me to spend more time at the church?"

Given the modal ages of CPSA survivors, if there were no intrapsychic conflicts prior to the abuse, child survivors would most likely be in the stage of becoming an "apprentice" in the world of work and school, seeking acceptance through competence and achievement, or of adolescent exploration of who he or she is apart from his or her parents. The need for affiliation and acceptance at the core of these stages makes the child particularly vulnerable to abuse and exploitation. Adult female survivors, on the other hand, would most likely be in one of two psychosocial stages. Young adults struggle to find a life partner and satisfying love relationship to balance the demands and tensions of work, while middle-aged adults struggle to feel that they are needed and have made a contribution to society. It is therefore notable that when the women in Flynn's (2000) dissertation study marked their CPSA experience as beginning in adulthood, they reported that their "affairs" with clergymen began in the context of increased activity in their religious communities due to either marital or occupational dissatisfaction. The clinical implications are striking. The adult female survivor's psychosocial developmental stage may strongly influence her attempt to make sense of the clergyperson's sexual violation by framing it as an "affair." Such framing is likely to obscure, erroneously, the egregious breach of fiduciary trust inherent in a clergyman raping or sexually abusing a woman who has sought his counsel.

What is notable about Erikson's developmental stages is that he also discussed the importance of culture and society to psychosocial development. In considering culture as a possible moderating psychosocial factor of CPSA, the literature raises a broader question about how culture should be defined. Kenny and McEachern (2000) extensively reviewed the empirical literature on ethnicity (White, Hispanic, Asian, and African American) and its potential role as a moderator in the incidence, prevalence, disclosure, and posttraumatic sequelae of CSA. Findings were mixed and contradictory, which the authors attributed to problems in sampling and sample size, operational definitions of key variables, and potentially real cultural differences in rates of disclosure and the expression of posttraumatic symptoms. A more recent study of the contribution of ethnicity to clinical presentation of domestic violence survivors controlled for confounding variables such as socioeconomic class and type of abuse and demonstrated that African-American women and Caucasian women had very different presentations (Torres, Harrington, Shipherd, & Resick, 2006). Caucasian women reported more symptoms of anxiety and dissociation, and had impaired self-reference, whereas African-American women reported higher levels of anger, irritability, and defensive avoidance. High rates of sexual and physical abuse were found in a small-sample qualitative study of Native-American women (Bohn, 2003), but these results will need considerable replication. More promising culture-related variables may be those pertaining to social learning: patriarchal attitudes toward women and children (Alaggia, 2001; Purvis & Ward, 2006), parental religiosity (Webb & Witmer, 2003), acceptance of violence, or the Asian idea of "saving face" (Hall, Teten, DeGarmo, Sue, & Stephens, 2005). There are no specific examinations of culture in CPSA and culture is only beginning to be addressed in the larger literature on recovery from abuse. We are hopeful that texts such as this one can assist researchers and clinicians by providing a conceptualization for their work with a goal of finding empirically supported treatments for survivors.

SUMMARY OF DEVELOPMENTAL FACTORS IN CPSA

In sum, knowing the age at which CPSA occurred can provide some insight into the idiographic problems a survivor may be experiencing in addition to posttraumatic symptomatology. Both adult and child survivors of CPSA describe the progression of the abusive relationship in similar ways, yet symptomatology varies greatly owing to the survivors' age, gender, and cognitive, emotional, and physical development. Culture and ethnicity may also play a role in how the survivor discusses the abuse and to whom he or she discloses, but the dearth of research findings in this area prevents us from knowing in what ways culture may serve as a potential moderator of recovery.

GENDER AS A MODERATING FACTOR IN CPSA

The NCSAR underscores that the proportion of male survivors of CPSA is unusually high compared to other sexual abuse survivor populations. Along similar lines, Disch and Avery (2001) surveyed 149 survivors of sexual abuse by clergy and medical and mental health professionals. The group of CPSA survivors had a significantly higher proportion of men ($n = 10/28$, 26.3%) than either survivors of abuse by medical ($n = 2/21$, 9.5%) or mental health professionals ($n = 6/90$, 6.7%). Males may constitute a particularly high risk group given that male CSA survivors typically hesitate to report their abuse as frequently as female survivors, thus perpetuating the secrecy in which the abusive relationship occurs (Bolton et al., 1989; Finkelhor, 1993; Lamb & Edgar-Smith, 1994). Some theorists speculate that this underreporting may be linked to male gender socialization, as articulated by Lew (1990): "Men are simply not supposed to be victimized. A 'real man' is expected to be able to protect himself in any situation. . . . When he experiences victimization, our culture expects him to be able to 'deal with it like a man'" (p. 41). Lew additionally suggested that signs of a male survivor's weakness (e.g., crying, trembling) is likely to provoke a violent response from the male perpetrator: "The behavior is considered weak and un-masculine, and becomes a justification for the adult's brutality" (p. 49). In the sample of male CPSA perpetrators surveyed by the NCSAR, 8% threatened violence, including physical threats with weapons, and 135 of the accused priests were alleged to have perpetrated extremely violent sexual acts (i.e., penetration with an object, group or coerced sex). Although these violent acts constituted less than 2% of alleged CPSA, a rate substantially lower than the 10%–25% reported by Holmes and Slap's (1998) review of the literature, it is notable that the majority of survivors of these extreme violations were boys (for penetration with an object, 61 boys versus 26 girls; for group or coerced sex, 47 boys versus 3 girls). This apparent gender-based discrepancy in the level of perpetrated violence may differentiate CPSA from other forms of abuse.

While we have been focusing on male perpetrators in this discussion, it is also important to recognize that gender of the perpetrator may also play a role in the victim's silence: "Abuse is typically perpetrated differently by a female and involves physical tenderness and physical and emotional seduction. The victim therefore may not be aware that what transpired was abusive" (Courtois, 1988, p. 284). Regardless of the type of abuse perpetrated, boys are less likely than girls to disclose abuse or admit that they have problems resulting from the abuse due to male socialization to be self-reliant and "tough" (Kia-Keating, Grossman, Sorsoli, & Epstein, 2005). However, boys are more likely to come to the attention of counselors indirectly due to extreme and aggressive acting out and self-injurious behaviors (Bolton et al., 1989; Garnefski & Diekstra, 1997; Holmes, Offen, & Waller, 1997; Holmes & Slap, 1998; Kendall-Tackett et al., 1993; Nielsen, 1983). In contrast, girls are more likely to report such problems as depression, anxiety, and general fear about safety (Feiring, Taska, & Lewis, 2002; Friedrich, 1996; Friedrich, Urquiza, & Beilke, 1986). Boys may demonstrate exaggerated displays of narcissistic rage and narcissistic invulnerability in defensive response to posttraumatic feelings of fear and vulnerability, whereas girls may become frightened at their own surges in rage and vengeful feelings (Pynoos & Nader, 1993). Gender-based disparities in symptom presentation and disclosure have been observed to persist into adulthood (Gold, Elhai, Lucenko, & Swingle, 1998; Heath, Bean, & Feinauer, 1996).

Differences in socialization about emotional awareness and expression also play an important role when assessing the effects of CPSA. To the extent that boys are at baseline more emotionally muted than girls (e.g., Casey, 1993), their CPSA–related distress may be harder to detect. Thus, they may "fly under the radar" of caring parents and professionals and inadvertently give the impression that they "weren't hurt that bad" by the abuse. For this reason, Bolton and colleagues (1989) advocated that helping professionals take a more proactive and assertive approach to getting boys suspected of being abused into treatment and not take their statements of being "fine" at face value.

Scholars in the psychology of women field have observed consistent differences in the ways that men and women relate to one another and to the outside world. The distinction has been characterized as a male "agentic" orientation toward dominance and self-assertion versus the female orientation toward "embeddedness" and "communion" with others (Chodorow, 1974); male self-centeredness versus female self-in-relation (Gilligan, 1982); and a male drive toward "separate self" versus a female drive toward "cognitive intersubjectivity" (Surrey, 1991). The core idea posed by these authors is that men generally feel most alive and competent when they are acting independently and women feel most alive and competent when they are in a mutually beneficial relationship (Chodorow, 1974). It is notable that the female survivors surveyed by Flynn (2000) and Fortune (1989) describe how the positive aspects of their pastoral counseling relationships facilitated the clergy-perpetrator's ability to coerce them into sexual activity but also created an uncomfortable feeling of dissonance.

The contrast between males' and females' relational orientation is quite striking when one compares their narratives in studies of CPSA. Whereas the autobiographical narratives of the male survivors focus exclusively on the theme of "what abuse did to me," "How I wish it could be different," and "How much I hate and want to exact revenge against my abuser" (Bera, 1995; Isely, 1996; Ponton & Goldstein, 2004), the female survivors' narratives report unwanted "obsession" with the perpetrator, even after the abuse (Flynn, 2000, pp. 138–139) and feelings of being "abandoned" and "betrayed" by the church after the abusive relationship was revealed (pp. 121–122). These thematic differences speak to different needs that adult CPSA survivors may wish to have fulfilled in therapy and by their social support systems. Male survivors may need to feel that their anger is justified and to mourn the loss of innocence and a carefree life. Female survivors may need to feel validated in their ambivalent feelings about their relationship with the perpetrator and church. This is not to say that males do not have needs to form intimate relationships with others or that females do not wish to assert themselves, but that knowledge of these gender-mediated relational issues can inform therapy beyond a PTSD diagnosis.

IMPLICATIONS FOR TREATMENT

There is hope for survivors of CPSA on several levels. First and foremost, changes in our cultural awareness of the problem may make disclosure easier for survivors than in years past when there was little recognition that CPSA occurred. Second, mental health treatment has been found to alleviate the symptoms of PTSD following other types of sexual abuse and has helped survivors to live fuller, more productive lives marked by improvements in both physical and mental health. Cognitive-behavioral treatment (CBT) for PTSD has thus far received the most empirical support for both adults (Bradley, Green, Russ, Dutra, & Westen, 2005; Rothbaum, Meadows, Resick, & Foy, 2000; van Etten & Taylor, 1998) and children and adolescents (Cohen, Berliner, & March, 2000; Finkelhor & Berliner, 1995). Commonly used CBT protocols include but are not limited to Cognitive Processing Therapy (CPT; Resick & Schnicke, 1993), Prolonged Exposure (Foa, Rothbaum, Riggs, & Murdock, 1991; Foa et al., 1999), and Stress Inoculation Training (Foa et al., 1991, 1999). Broadly speaking, CBT for PTSD includes the following components: psychoeducation about PTSD for clients and their significant others (e.g., spouses, parents, and teachers); cognitive restructuring to address self-blaming and depressive thoughts; anxiety management to address hyperarousal symptoms; behavioral exposure to address avoidance symptoms; and imaginal exposure to disarm the haunting and intrusive power of the trauma itself. Several controlled trials have demonstrated the effectiveness of CBT, as compared with other interventions and wait-list control in survivors of CSA and adult assault survivors (Cloitre, Koenen, Cohen, & Han, 2002; Resick et al., 2002; Resick & Schnicke, 1992). For overwhelming arousal symptoms and nightmares, pharmacotherapy can also be helpful (Friedman, Davidson, Mellman, & Southwick, 2000). Creative arts therapies are additionally recommended for children and highly dissociative adults who are not verbally skilled or are uncomfortable describing their traumas in words, or conversely for highly intellectualized clients who have difficulty accessing their emotions (Johnson, 2000).

Clients can usually tolerate traditional CBT therapy, including the psychoeducation, cognitive reprocessing, and imaginal and behavioral exposure components. Outcomes are particularly favorable in cases of isolated incidents of rape, when there is no evidence of chronic abuse or psychopathology, and when there is good social support (Meadows & Foa, 1998). However, even when these elements are not present, as in the case for the majority of CPSA survivors, therapy can still be effective. For example, CBT for PTSD has been shown to be effective in the presence of significant mental health comorbidities (Blanchard et al., 2003; Paunovic & Öst, 2001) and when it is administered many years after the development of symptoms (Resick et al., 2002). In fact, the benefits of PTSD treatment have even been shown to have favorable effect on comorbid physical problems, including chronic pain (Shipherd, Beck, Hamblen, Lackner, & Freeman, 2003; Shipherd et al., 2007) and overutilization of health care (Shipherd et al., 2006), in addition to reducing guilt-related cognitions (Resick et al., 2002).

To manage more complex symptoms, these evidence-based treatments are often supplemented with other CBT–based interventions. For example, some CPSA survivors may be referred to Dialectical Behavior Therapy (DBT; Linehan, 1993) or to a Skills Training in Affect and Interpersonal Regulation–model treatment (STAIR; Cloitre et al., 2002), where affect regulation and interpersonal effectiveness skills can be added to the PTSD treatment. Similarly, substance abusers may be referred to a Seeking Safety (Najavits, 2002) program to learn to deal with PTSD and substance abuse issues simultaneously. These treatments also have empirical support and may be particularly beneficial for those who find that the most disruptive symptoms they experience are in these areas of interpersonal effectiveness, emotional dysregulation, or substance abuse.

Significant others have an important role to play in the treatment of these conditions (see Wind, Sullivan, & Levins, 2008). Research has shown that high levels of expressed criticism, hostility, and emotional overinvolvement in the families of adults and children with a wide range of medical and psychiatric disorders, including PTSD, are highly predictive of psychiatric relapse and worse behavioral therapy outcome (Wearden, Tarrier, Barrowclough, Zastony, & Rahill, 2000). This line of research has impelled the development of very successful psychoeducational treatments targeted at lowering families' negative expressed emotion and teaching constructive communication and problem-solving skills, thereby producing better outcomes for identified patients (see McFarlane, 2002 for review). Dickstein, Hinz, and Eth (1991) outlined helpful psychoeducational techniques to use with families following extrafamilial and intrafamilial sexual abuse, both of which may be applicable to the unique situation of a perpetrating clergyman. Family members can also be engaged as helpful partners in cognitive-behavioral skill building, as has been shown in the families of patients with severe anxiety disorders (see Steketee & Fogler, 2005 for review).

SPECIAL CONSIDERATIONS FOR THE TREATMENT OF CPSA SURVIVORS

In this article, we consider CPSA to be similar to incest and other forms of sexual abuse in which the perpetrator has been a parental figure, family member, or a member of a profession falling under Bonosky's (1995) definition of fiduciary responsibility. As has been noted earlier, such traumas can result in various outcomes, including chronic and severe symptoms of complex PTSD and a damaged sense of spirituality and connection with one's God and church. To the extent that CPSA survivors follow this trajectory (Bera, 1995; Isely, 1996), it is imperative that behavioral scientists join with pastoral and mental health counselors to study the mechanisms central to recovery and develop effective, empirically supported interventions.

While there are studies demonstrating that CBT can be effective even for clients who present with complex PTSD (Resick, Nishith, & Griffin, 2003), some survivors will require additional intervention. We view the theories of gender and development discussed in this paper to be helpful lenses for understanding how these survivors may present in therapy. For example, an adult who was abused as a child may be experiencing unresolved psychosocial crises and have trauma-related thoughts that are more developmentally appropriate for the age at which the abuse occurred. Experiencing dissonance between a survivor's appearance and their behavior is common: we expect adults to "act their age," and when there are clear physical markers of development and when those markers generally correspond to increasing cognitive sophistication, it seems self-evident that a prepubertal and a postpubertal child would experience trauma differently.

We are not proposing that pastoral counselors and mental health professionals need to be experts in developmental psychology to be able to help CPSA survivors, but we do encourage providers to recognize that an adult client may present with issues that are developmentally similar to preadolescent children. Clues that this may be the case include abuse history (i.e., reporting that abuse occurred during childhood or adolescence), the client voicing concerns about identity or competence that sound more developmentally appropriate for an earlier life stage, or difficulty thinking abstractly or taking another's point of view in the absence of measurable cognitive impairment. In very extreme cases of complex PTSD, the client may actually present with a younger dissociative persona (Chu, 1998; Herman, 1992).

The Eriksonian stages of psychosocial development described earlier may be particularly difficult for altar boys who are abused by male clerics, particularly in religions where homosexuality is viewed as a sin. Altar boys are in the bind of being apprenticed to the church, most likely to become an active member of the Christian community, and perhaps even to become a clergyman (e.g., Isely, 1996), yet are being abused in secret by their highly regarded mentors. Erikson also noted that adolescents are often keenly reactive to their peers' approval, and one can only imagine the burden a young adolescent male would experience facing his friends with the "double stigma" of being not only a survivor, but a survivor of (in the imagined eyes of his friends) "homosexual" CPSA (Finkelhor, 1986; Pierce & Pierce, 1985). Indeed, research suggests that sexually abused boys commonly report confusion and anxiety about sexual orientation in reaction to CSA (Ponton & Goldstein, 2004; Rogers & Terry, 1984, in Isley & Isley, 1990).

Depression, self-doubt, and guilt are often stumbling blocks to disclosing the abuse and accessing treatment. Furthermore, societal reactions will often vary, with many community members who may share the survivor's erroneous beliefs about their sharing responsibility for the CPSA, thereby decreasing social support in the survivor's time of need. A clear example of this type of complicated presentation would be a woman who describes "having an affair" with her priest. This statement could be taken at face value by a therapist who assumes a relationship between two consulting adults. Unfortunately, for many adult women who are survivors of CPSA the ability to name what has happened to them and to heal from it is taken away by minimizing the experience and calling it simply "an affair" rather than acknowledging the inherent power differential between a cleric and parishioner. However, without considering this experience as CPSA, the survivor's resulting symptoms of depression, anxiety (including PTSD), and low self-esteem may be difficult to understand. Thoughts such as "I tempted him into an affair when I went to him for advice on my marriage" may be present and could be addressed by a mental health professional who is prepared to consider the relationship dynamics between a priest and his congregation.

Thoburn and Whitman's (2004) anonymous nationwide survey of protestant ministers found that ministers who endorsed their own marital infidelity tended on average to have affairs with church members and staff rather than with people outside the church. For our purposes, we consider this a case of CPSA where the minister utilizes his or her role in the church to gain access to a sexual partner. This type of CPSA is particularly insidious and perhaps more difficult to disclose, because many survivors of this type of abuse may not recognize that the unequal balance of power made them much more vulnerable than they would have been otherwise. For many women who have survived this type of abuse, it is likely that they will feel complicit in the abuse by stating that they are "old enough to have said no." However, what many of these CPSA survivors fail to recognize is that the power dynamics inherent in a counseling relationship diminish a person's capacity to refuse sexual advances (Disch & Avery, 2001; Underwood, 2002). To the extent that family and religious community members hold the survivor responsible for their traumas, thereby adding to survivors' distress, psychoeducational groups of the type described in the previous section may help them tailor their reactions and create a more constructive, healing environment to facilitate recovery.

While no randomized controlled trials have been conducted with survivors of CPSA, it is likely that the extant literature on recovery from CSA and sexual assault can be a useful starting point. It is likely that at some point in the future, a treatment package may be developed that is specific to treating PTSD symptoms and the spiritual/existential disruptions that occur following CPSA. One promising treatment, *Solace for the Soul*, is designed to help repair CPSA survivors' sense of spiritual well-being and connection to God (Murray-Swank & Pargament, 2005). We would hope to see the spiritual elements of this treatment combined with what we know to be effective for treating PTSD. However, to date there is no literature to guide clinicians with this difficult task aside from those treatments discussed previously (e.g., DBT, STAIR, Seeking Safety) that address equally difficult, albeit different, presentations of survivors.

DISCUSSION AND FUTURE DIRECTIONS

In summary, our knowledge of the effects of CPSA is still in its infancy. More research is clearly needed to begin to more fully appreciate the experiences of survivors and to understand the best methods of treatment after this abuse. What we do know is that there are a wide range of experiences that are captured under the umbrella term of CPSA, including assaults on men and women of all ages who experience the abuse differently. On the whole, we believe that CPSA is fundamentally an abuse of power that is complicated by the perpetrator's role as a spiritual leader. For those who have survived this abuse, we have trust in the mental health community's ability to address the symptoms of PTSD they commonly face. At this time, we know of one intervention for the impact that CPSA can have on religious faith or spirituality (Murray-Swank & Pargament, 2005), but no treatments that combine spiritual and cognitive-behavioral approaches to symptom reduction. Currently, we know very little about factors relevant to disclosure of CPSA, psychological symptoms in the aftermath of CPSA, the effect of culture, social learning variables, or gene-environment interactions (Moffitt, Caspi, & Rutter, 2006) that could explain the different pathways of recovery. Clearly, systematic study of the problem of CPSA and recovery in its aftermath are warranted if we are to develop evidence-based interventions for CPSA survivors.

As recognition of CPSA continues to grow, we are hopeful that all survivors, regardless of gender or age, will find acceptance and be able to access treatment when needed. For therapists who work with survivors, we strongly encourage consideration of developmental factors and gender-specific issues in the assessment, case formulation, and treatment plan. Our review suggests that survivors of CPSA are a heterogeneous population, and "one-size fits all" treatments, even those that are targeted at complex symptom presentations, will be insufficient to help their recovery. It is not enough to know whether a survivor is distressed. Our review suggests that it will be equally, if not more, important to know what aspects of the survivor's experience are perceived to be distressing based on his or her stages of cognitive and psychosocial development as well as gender-mediated relational orientation.

In conclusion, we offer an aspirational goal for our colleagues: a dramatic increase in the research and development of treatments for CPSA. Toward this end, we recommend the development of a treatment that is able to address survivors' developmental needs and gender-specific concerns while simultaneously encouraging their spiritual growth and healing.

NOTES

1. Given this finding, it is important to note that 5% of the female child survivors of CPSA surveyed for the NCSAR also reported that they were threatened with a weapon.

2. However, other CPSA–specific symptoms noted by Farrell and Taylor are more anxiety-based and probably generalize across age (e.g., inability to engage in sacraments, difficulty praying).

REFERENCES

Alaggia, R. (2001). Cultural and religious influences in maternal response to intrafamilial child sexual abuse: Charting new territory for research and treatment. *Journal of Child Sexual Abuse, 10*, 41–60.

American Psychiatric Association. (2000). *Diagnostic and statistical manual of mental disorders* (4th ed., text rev.). Washington DC: Author.

Bera, W. H. (1995). *Clergy sexual abuse and male survivors: A study of stress and coping among 25 men abused by the same minister during their adolescence.* Unpublished doctoral dissertation, University of Minnesota, Minneapolis, MN.

Blanchard, E. B., Hickling, E. J., Devineni, T., Veazey, C. H., Galovski, T. E., Mundy, E., et al. (2003). A controlled evaluation of cognitive behavioral therapy for posttraumatic stress in motor vehicle accident survivors. *Behaviour Research and Therapy, 41,* 79–96.

Bohn, D. K. (2003). Lifetime physical and sexual abuse, substance abuse, depression, and suicide attempts among Native American women. *Issues in Mental Health Nursing, 24,* 333–352.

Bolton, F. G., Jr., Morris, L. A., & MacEachron, A. E. (1989). *Males at risk: The other side of child sexual abuse.* Newbury Park, CA: Sage Publications.

Bonosky, N. (1995). Boundary violations in social work supervision: Clinical, educational, and legal implications. *The Clinical Supervisor, 13,* 79–95.

Bradley, R., Greene, J., Russ, E., Dutra, L., & Westen, D. (2005). A multidimensionl meta-analysis of psychotherapy for PTSD. *American Journal of Psychiatry, 162,* 214–227.

Brooks-Gunn, J. (1991). How stressful is the transition to adolescence for girls? In M. E. Colten & S. Gore (Eds.), *Adolescent stress: Causes and consequences* (pp. 131–149). New York: Aldine De Gruyter.

Casey, R. (1993). Children's emotional experience: Relations among expression, self-report, and understanding. *Developmental Psychology, 29,* 119–129.

Celenza, A. (2004). Sexual misconduct in the clergy: The search for the Father. *Studies in Gender and Sexuality, 5,* 213–232.

Chodorow, N. (1974). Family structure and feminine personality. In M. Z. Rosaldo & L. Lamphere (Eds.), *Women, culture, and society* (pp. 81–105). Stanford, CA: Stanford University Press.

Christian Ethics Today: Journal of Christian Ethics. (2000, October). Special issue on clergy sexual abuse. Retrieved April 13, 2005, from www.christianethicstoday.com.

Chu, J. A. (1998). *Rebuilding shattered lives: The responsible treatment of complex post-traumatic and dissociative disorders.* New York: John Wiley & Sons.

Cicchetti, D., & Lynch, M. (1993). Toward an ecological/transactional model of community violence and child maltreatment: Consequences for children's development. *Psychiatry, 56,* 96–118.

Cloitre, M., Koenen, K. C., Cohen, L. R., & Han, H. (2002). Skills training in affective and interpersonal regulation followed by exposure: A phase-based treatment for PTSD related to childhood abuse. *Journal of Consulting and Clinical Psychology, 70*(5), 1067–1074.

Cohen, J. A., Berliner, L., & March, J. S. (2000). Treatment of children and adolescents. In E. Foa, T. Keane, & M. Friedman (Eds.), *Effective treatments for PTSD* (pp. 106–138). New York: Guilford Press.

Courtois, C. A. (1988). *Healing the incest wound: Adult survivors in therapy.* New York: W. W. Norton & Company.

Desai, S., Arias, I., Thompson, M. P., & Basile, K. C. (2002). Childhood victimization and subsequent adult revictimization assessed in a nationally representative sample of women and men. *Violence and Victims, 17*(6), 639–653.

Dickstein, L. J., Hinz, L. D., & Eth, S. (1991). Treatment of sexually abused children and adolescents. In A. Tasman & S. M. Goldfinger (Eds.), *American Psychiatric Press review of psychiatry* (Vol. 10, pp. 345–366). Washington, DC: American Psychiatric Association.

Disch, E., & Avery, N. (2001). Sex in the consulting room, the examining room, and the sacristy: Survivors of sexual abuse by professionals. *American Journal of Orthopsychiatry, 71*(2), 204–217.

Duncan, D. F. (1996). Growing up under the gun: Children and adolescents coping with violent neighborhoods. *Journal of Primary Prevention, 16,* 343–356.

Erikson, E. H. (1950/1985). *Childhood and society* (35th anniversary ed.). New York: Wiley.

Farrell, D. P., & Taylor, M. (1999). Sexual abuse by clergy and the implications for survivors. *Changes—An International Journal of Psychology and Psychotherapy, 17*(1), 52–59.

Farrell, D. P., & Taylor, M. (2000). Silenced by God: An examination of unique characteristics within sexual abuse by clergy. *Counselling Psychology Review, 15*(1), 22–31.

Feiring, C., Taska, L., & Lewis, M. (2002). Adjustment following sexual abuse discovery: The role of shame and attributional style. *Developmental Psychology, 38,* 79–82.

Felitti, V. S. (1991). Long term medical consequences of incest, rape and molestation. *Southern Medical Journal, 84*(3), 328–331.

Finkelhor, D. (1986). *A sourcebook on child sexual abuse.* Beverly Hills, CA: Sage Publications.

Finkelhor, D. (1993). Epidemiological factors in the clinical identification of child sexual abuse. *Child Abuse and Neglect, 17,* 67–70.

Finkelhor, D., & Berliner, L. (1995). Research on the treatment of sexually abused children: A review and recommendations. *Journal of the American Academy of Child and Adolescent Psychiatry, 34*(11), 1408–1423.

Fishburn, J. (1982). Male clergy adultery as vocational confusion. *Christian Century,* 922.

Flynn, K. A. (2000). *Clergy sexual abuse of women: A specialized form of trauma.* Unpublished doctoral dissertation, Claremont Graduate University, Claremont, California.

Foa, E. B., Dancu, C. V., Hembree, E. A., Jaycox, L. H., Meadows, E. A., & Street, G. P. (1999). A comparison of exposure therapy, stress inoculation training, and their combination for reducing post-traumatic stress disorder in female assault victims. *Journal of Consulting and Clinical Psychology, 67*(2), 194–200.

Foa, E. B., Rothbaum, B. O., Riggs, D. S., & Murdock, T. B. (1991). Treatment of post-traumatic stress disorder in rape victims: A comparison between cognitive-behavioral procedures and counseling. *Journal of Consulting and Clinical Psychology, 59*(5), 715–723.

Fogler, J. M., Shipherd, J. C., Rowe, E., Jensen, J., & Clarke, S. (2008). A theoretical foundation for understanding clergy-perpetrated sexual abuse. *Journal of Child Sexual Abuse, 17*(3–4), 301–328.

Fortune, M. (1989). *Is nothing sacred? When sex invades the pastoral relationship.* San Francisco: Harper & Row.

Franz, T. (2002). Power, patriarchy, and sexual abuse in the Christian church. *Traumatology, 8*, 1–12.

Friedman, M. J., Davidson, J. R., Mellman, T. A., & Southwick, S. M. (2000). Pharmacotherapy. In E. Foa, T. Keane, & M. Friedman (Eds.), *Effective treatments for PTSD* (pp. 84–105). New York: Guilford Press.

Friedrich, W. N. (1996). An integrated model of psychotherapy for abused children. In J. N. Briere, L. Berliner, J. A. Bulkley, C. Jenny, & T. Reid (Eds.), *The APSAC handbook on child maltreatment* (1st ed., pp. 104–118). Thousand Oaks, CA: Sage Publications.

Friedrich, W. N., Urquiza, A. J., & Beilke, R. L. (1986). Behavior problems in sexually abused young children. *Journal of Pediatric Psychology, 11*(1), 47–57.

Garnefski, N., & Diekstra, R. F. W. (1997). Child sexual abuse and emotional and behavioral problems in adolescence: Gender differences. *Journal of the American Academy of Child and Adolescent Psychiatry, 36*(3), 323–329.

Gilligan, C. (1982). *In a different voice*. Cambridge, MA: Harvard University Press.

Gold, S. N., Elhai, J. D., Lucenko, B. A., & Swingle, J. M. (1998). Abuse characteristics among childhood sexual abuse survivors in therapy: A gender comparison. *Child Abuse and Neglect, 22*, 1005–1012.

Golding, J. M. (1994). Sexual assault history and physical health in randomly selected Los Angeles women. *Health Psychology, 13*, 130–138.

Graber, J. A., & Brooks-Gunn, J. (1996). Transitions and turning points: Navigating the passage from childhood to adolescence. *Developmental Psychology, 32*, 768–776.

Hall, G. C. N., Teten, A. L., DeGarmo, D. S., Sue, S., & Stephens, K. A. (2005). Ethnicity, culture, and sexual aggression: Risk and protective factors. *Journal of Consulting and Clinical Psychology, 73*, 830–840.

Hardman-Cromwell, Y. (1991). Power and sexual abuse in ministry. *Journal of Religious Thought, 1*, 65–72.

Harned, M. S. (2004). Does it matter what you call it? The relationship between labeling unwanted sexual experiences and distress. *Journal of Consulting and Clinical Psychology, 72*, 1090–1099.

Harter, S., & Buddin, B. J. (1987). Children's understanding of the simultaneity of two emotions: A five-stage developmental acquisition sequence. *Developmental Psychology, 23*, 388–399.

Heath, V., Bean, R., & Feinauer, L. (1996). Severity of childhood sexual abuse: Symptom differences between men and women. *American Journal of Family Therapy, 24*, 305–314.

Herman, J. (1992). *Trauma and recovery: The aftermath of violence—From domestic abuse to political terror*. New York: Basic Books.

Herman, J. L., Russell, D. E. H., & Trocki, K. (1986). Long-term effects of incestuous abuse in childhood. *American Journal of Psychiatry, 143*(10), 1293–1296.

Hetherington, E. M., & Parke, R. D. (1993). *Child psychology: A contemporary viewpoint* (4th ed.). New York: McGraw-Hill.

Holmes, G. R., Offen, L., & Waller, G. (1997). See no evil, hear no evil, speak no evil: Why do relatively few male victims of childhood sexual abuse receive help for abuse-related issues in adulthood? *Clinical Psychology Review, 17*(1), 69–88.

Holmes, W. C., & Slap, G. B. (1998). Sexual abuse of boys: Definition, prevalence, correlates, sequelae, and management. *Journal of the American Medical Association, 280*(21), 1855–1862.

Isely, P. J. (1996). *In their own voices: A qualitative study of men sexually abused as children by catholic clergy.* Unpublished doctoral dissertation, Boston University School of Education, Boston, Massachusetts.

Isely, P. J., & Isely, P. (1990). The sexual abuse of male children by church personnel: Intervention and prevention. *Pastoral Psychology, 39*(2), 85–99.

The John Jay College Research Team. (2004, February 27). *The nature and scope of the problem of sexual abuse of minors by Catholic priests and deacons in the United States: A research study conducted by the John Jay College of Criminal Justice (National Clergy Sex Abuse Report).* Retrieved April 13, 2005, from www.jjay.cuny.edu/churchstudy/main.asp.

Johnson, D. R. (2000). Creative therapies. In E. Foa, T. Keane, & M. Friedman (Eds.), *Effective treatments for PTSD* (pp. 302–314). New York: Guilford Press.

Keane, T. M., & Barlow, D. H. (2002). Post-traumatic stress disorder. In D. Barlow (Ed.), *Anxiety and its disorders: The nature and treatment of anxiety and panic* (2nd ed., pp. 418–453). New York: Guilford Press.

Keane, T. M., Weathers, F. W., & Foa, E. B. (2000). Diagnosis and assessment. In E. Foa, T. Keane, & M. Friedman (Eds.), *Effective treatments for PTSD* (pp. 18–36). New York: Guilford Press.

Kendall-Tackett, K. A., Williams, L. M., & Finkelhor, D. (1993). Impact of sexual abuse on children: A review and synthesis of recent empirical studies. *Psychological Bulletin, 113*(1), 164–180.

Kenny, M. C., & McEachern, A. G. (2000). Racial, ethnic, and cultural factors of childhood sexual abuse: A selected review of the literature. *Clinical Psychology Review, 20*, 905–922.

Kessler, B. L., & Bieschke, K. J. (1999). A retrospective analysis of shame, dissociation, and adult victimization in survivors of childhood sexual abuse. *Journal of Consulting and Clinical Psychology, 46*, 335–341.

Kessler, R. C., Sonnega, A., Bromet, E., Hughes, M., & Nelson, C. B. (1995). Post-traumatic stress disorder in the National Comorbidity Survey. *Archives of General Psychiatry, 52*, 1048–1060.

Kia-Keating, M., Grossman, F. K., Sorsoli, L., & Epstein, M. (2005). Containing and resisting masculinity: Narratives of renegotiation among resilient male survivors of childhood sexual abuse. *Psychology of Men & Masculinity, 6*, 169–185.

Lamb, S., & Edgar-Smith, S. (1994). Aspects of disclosure mediators of outcome of childhood sexual abuse. *Journal of Interpersonal Violence, 9*, 307–326.

Lew, M. (1990). *Victims no longer: Men recovering from incest and other sexual child abuse.* New York: Harper Collins.

Linehan, M. M. (1993). *Cognitive-behavioral treatment of borderline personality disorder.* New York: Guilford Press.

Lothstein, L. M. (2002). Treating clergy who sexually abuse minors: A 16-year experience in the Professionals and Clergy Program at the IOL. *Connecticut Psychologist, 56*, 1, 4.

Lovett, B. B. (2004). Child sexual abuse disclosure: Maternal response and other variables impacting the victim. *Child and Adolescent Social Work Journal, 21*, 355–371.

Maker, A. H., Kemmelmeier, M., & Peterson, C. (2001). Child sexual abuse, peer sexual abuse, and sexual assault in adulthood: A multi-risk model of revictimization. *Journal of Traumatic Stress, 14*, 351–368.

Marx, B. P., Heidt, J. M., & Gold, S. D. (2005). Perceived uncontrollability and unpredictability, self-regulation, and revictimization. *Review of General Psychology, 9*, 67–90.

McFarlane, W. R. (2002). *Multifamily groups in the treatment of severe psychiatric disorders*. New York: Guilford.

McLaughlin, B. R. (1994). Devastated spirituality: The impact of clergy sexual abuse on the survivor's relationship with God and the Church. *Sexual Addiction and Compulsivity, 1*, 145–158.

Meadows, E. A., & Foa, E. B. (1998). Intrusion, arousal, and avoidance: Sexual trauma survivors. In V. M. Follette, J. I. Ruzek, & F. R. Abueg (Eds.), *Cognitive-behavioral therapies for trauma* (pp. 100–123). New York: Guilford.

Mennen, F. E. (1993). Evaluation of risk factors in childhood sexual abuse. *Journal of the American Academy of Child and Adolescent Psychiatry, 32*, 934–939.

Moffitt, T. E., Caspi, A., & Rutter, M. (2006). Measured gene-environment interactions in psychopathology: Concepts, research strategies, and implications for research, intervention, and public understanding of genetics. *Perspectives on Psychological Science, 1*, 5–27.

Murray-Swank, N. A., & Pargament, K. I. (2005). God, where are you? Evaluating a spiritually-integrated intervention for sexual abuse. *Mental Health, Religion, & Culture, 8*, 191–203.

Najavits, L. M. (2002). *Seeking safety: A treatment manual for PTSD and substance abuse*. New York: Guilford Press.

Neustein, A., & Lesher, M. (2008). A single-case study of rabbinic sexual abuse in the orthodox Jewish community. *Journal of Child Sexual Abuse, 17*(3–4), 270–289.

Nielsen, T. (1983, November). Sexual abuse of boys: Current perspectives. *Personnel and Guidance Journal*, 139–142.

Norris, F. H., Foster, J. D., & Weisshaar, D. L. (2002). The epidemiology of sex differences in PTSD across developmental societal and research contexts. In R. Kimerling, P. Ouimette, & J. Wolfe (Eds.), *Gender and PTSD* (pp. 3–42). New York: Guilford Press.

Osofsky, J. D., & Scheeringa, M. S. (1997). Community and domestic violence exposure: Effects on development and psychopathology. In D. Cicchetti & S.Toth (Eds.), *Rochester Symposium on developmental psychopathology*, (Vol. 8: *Developmental perspectives on trauma: Theory, research, and intervention*, pp. 155–180). Rochester, NY: University of Rochester Press.

Paunovic, N., & Öst, L. G. (2001). Cognitive-behavior therapy vs exposure therapy in the treatment of PTSD in refugees. *Behaviour Research and Therapy, 39*, 1183–1197.

Pierce, R., & Pierce, L. H. (1985). The sexually abused child: A comparison of male and female victims. *Child Abuse and Neglect, 9*(2), 191–199.

Ponton, L., & Goldstein, D. (2004). Sexual abuse of boys by clergy. *Adolescent Psychiatry: Developmental and Clinical Studies, 28*, 209–229.

Pope, K. S., Levenson, H., & Schover, L. R. (1979). Sexual intimacy in psychology training: Results and implications of a national survey. *American Psychologist, 34*, 692–689.

Pope, K. S., Schover, L. R., & Levenson, H. (1980). Sexual behavior between clinical supervisors and trainees: Implications for professional standards. *Professional Psychology, 11*, 157–162.

Purvis, M., & Ward, T. (2006). The role of culture in understanding child sexual offending: Examining feminist perspectives. *Aggression and Violent Behavior, 11*, 298–312.

Pynoos, R. S., & Nader, K. (1993). Issues in the treatment of post-traumatic stress in children and adolescents. In J. P. Wilson & B. Raphael (Eds.), *International handbook of traumatic stress syndromes* (pp. 535–549). New York: Plenum Press.

Resick, P. A., & Calhoun, K. S. (2001). Post-traumatic stress disorder. In D. Barlow (Ed.), *Clinical handbook of psychological disorders: A step-by-step treatment manual* (3rd ed., pp. 60–113). New York: Guilford Press.

Resick, P. A., Nishith, P., & Griffin, M. G. (2003). How well does cognitive-behavioral therapy treat symptoms of complex PTSD? An examination of child sexual abuse survivors within a clinical trial. *CNS Spectrums, 8*, 340–355.

Resick, P. A., Nishith, P., Weaver, T. L., Astin, M. C., & Feuer, C. A. (2002). A comparison of cognitive-processing therapy with prolonged exposure and a waiting condition for the treatment of chronic posttraumatic stress disorder in female rape victims. *Journal of Consulting and Clinical Psychology, 70*(4), 867–879.

Resick, P. A., & Schnicke, M. K. (1992). Cognitive processing therapy for sexual assault victims. *Journal of Consulting and Clinical Psychology, 60*(5), 748–756.

Resick, P. A., & Schnicke, M. K. (1993). *Cognitive processing therapy for rape victims: A treatment manual.* Newbury Park, CA: Sage Publications.

Rheingold, A. A., Acierno, R., & Resnick, H. S. (2004). Trauma, post-traumatic stress disorder, and health risk behaviors. In P. P. Schnurr & B. L. Green (Eds.), *Trauma and health: Physical health consequences of exposure to extreme stress* (pp. 217–243). Washington, DC: American Psychological Association.

Rogers, C. M., & Terry, T. (1984). Clinical intervention with boy victims of sexual abuse. In I. R. Stuart & J. G. Greer (Eds.), *Victims of sexual aggression: Treatment of children, women, and men* (pp. 91–104). New York: Van Nostrand Reinhold.

Rothbaum, B. O., Meadows, E. A., Resick, P., & Foy, D. W. (2000). Cognitive-behavioral therapy. In E. Foa, T. Keane, & M. Friedman (Eds.), *Effective treatments for PTSD* (pp. 60–83). New York: Guilford Press.

Ruzek, J. I., Polusny, R. A., & Abueg, F. R. (1998). Assessment and treatment of concurrent post-traumatic stress disorder and substance abuse. In V. M. Follette, J. I. Ruzek, & F. R. Abueg (Eds.), *Cognitive-behavioral therapies for trauma* (pp. 226–255). New York: Guilford Press.

Salter, A. C. (1992). Epidemiology of child sexual abuse. In W. O'Donohue & J. Greer (Eds.), *The sexual abuse of children: Theory and research* (pp. 108–138). Hillsdale, NJ: Erlbaum.

Schnurr, P. P., & Jankowski, M. K. (1999). Physical health and post-traumatic stress disorder: Review and synthesis. *Seminars in Clinical Neuropsychiatry, 4*(4), 295–304.

Shipherd, J. C., Beck, J. G., Hamblen, J. L., Lackner, J. M., & Freeman, J. B. (2003). A preliminary examination of treatment for posttraumatic stress disorder in chronic pain patients: A case study. *Journal of Traumatic Stress, 16*(5), 451–457.

Shipherd, J. C., Keyes, M., Jovanovic, T., Gordon-Brown, V., Ready, D., Baltzell, D., et al. (2006). *Effects of PTSD treatment on health care utilization behavior.* Unpublished manuscript.

Shipherd, J. C., Keyes, M., Jovanovic, T., Ready, D., Baltzell, D., Worley, V., et al. (2007). Veterans seeking treatment for posttraumatic stress disorder: What about comorbid chronic pain? *Journal of Rehabilitation Research and Development, 44*(2), 153–165.

Shipherd, J. C., Stafford, J., & Tanner, L. R. (2005). Predicting alcohol and drug abuse in Persian Gulf War veterans: What role do PTSD symptoms play? *Addictive Behaviors, 30*, 595–599.

Somer, E., & Szwarcberg, S. (2001). Variables in delayed disclosure of childhood sexual abuse. *American Journal of Orthopsychiatry, 71*, 332–341.

Steketee, G., & Fogler, J. (2005). The family of a patient with a severe anxiety disorder. In N. Sartorius, J. Leff, J. J. Lopez-Ibor, M. Maj, & A. Okasha (Eds.) *Families and mental disorders: From burden to empowerment* (pp. 87–112). Chichester, England: Wiley & Sons.

Surrey, J. (1991). The self-in-relation: A theory of women's development. In J. Jordan, A. Kaplan, J. B. Miller, A. Stiver, & J. Surrey (Eds.), *Women's growth in connection: Writings from the Stone Center* (pp. 51–66). New York: Guilford Press.

Terr, L. C. (1991). Childhood traumas: An outline and overview. *American Journal of Psychiatry, 148*, 10–20.

Thoburn, J., & Whitman, M. (2004). Clergy affairs: Emotional investment, longevity of relationship and affair partners. *Pastoral Psychology, 52*(6), 491–506.

Torres, S., Harrington, E., Shipherd, J. C., & Resick, P. A. (2006). *Race and battered women: Differences in PTSD and other trauma-related symptoms.* Unpublished manuscript.

Underwood, A. (2002). *Abuse of power as a justice issue.* Retrieved May 17, 2005, from www.votf.org/papers/AbuseofPowerasjusticeissue.html.

van Etten, M. L., & Taylor, S. (1998). Comparative efficacy of treatments for PTSD: A meta-analysis. *Clinical Psychology and Psychotherapy, 5*(3), 126–145.

Wagner, A. W., & Linehan, M. M. (1998). Dissociative behavior. In V. M. Follette, J. I. Ruzek, & F. R. Abueg (Eds.), *Cognitive-behavioral therapies for trauma* (pp. 191–225). New York: Guilford Press.

Wearden, A. J., Tarrier, N., Barrowclough, C., Zastowny, T. R., & Rahill, A. A. (2000). A review of expressed emotion research in healthcare. *Clinical Psychology Review, 20*, 633–666.

Webb, M., & Whitmer, K. J. O. (2003). Parental religiosity, abuse history, and maintenance of beliefs taught in the family. *Mental Health, Religion, & Culture, 6*, 229–239.

Wind, L. H., Sullivan, J. M., & Levins, D. J. (2008). Survivors' perspectives on the impact of clergy sexual abuse on families of origin. *Journal of Child Sexual Abuse, 17*(3–4), 238–254.

World Health Organization. (2001, May). *Gender disparities in mental health.* Paper presented at the Ministerial Round Tables of the 54th World Health Assembly, Geneva, Switzerland.

The Impact of Sexual Abuse on Sexual Identity Formation in Gay Men

Stephen Brady

The pernicious impact of sexual abuse on child development has been well documented. Herman (1992) stated, "Repeated trauma in adult life erodes the structure of the personality already formed, but repeated trauma in childhood forms and deforms the personality" (p. 96). She emphasized how exposure to early trauma disempowers the child and contributes to a disconnection from others, often leading to distrust, shame, guilt, inferiority, confusion, isolation, and despair. Current thinking (Doyle, 2003) regarding clergy-perpetrated sexual abuse (CPSA) suggests its impact is similar to familial incest, which has a particularly devastating impact on identity development (see also Fogler, Shipherd, Clarke, Jensen, & Rowe, 2008). Factors that support this comparison include the following: the families of many victims were closely allied with the life of their church—a spiritual family; the abuse tended to occur over an extended period of time, similar to many cases of incest; adults frequently did not believe reports of abuse when alerted to it, which often also occurs in cases of incest; church leaders tried to silence victims to avoid scandal, also a repeated theme in incest; and many victims did not disclose the abuse until adulthood, again similar to many cases of incest (Doyle, 2003).

This article examines the incidence of childhood physical and sexual abuse in the lives of gay men and extrapolates from these findings to the probable impact of CPSA for this group. It will posit a process of normative gay identity formation and address the impact of abuse on this process. The author will also make detailed recommendations for mental health clinicians treating gay men who have been abused and present two case vignettes. It should be noted that lesbians have a parallel process of identity development that can also be negatively influenced by abuse. However, the issues of lesbian development and abuse are beyond the scope of this article.

ABUSE IN THE LIVES OF GAY MEN

Emerging data suggests that gay males have an increased risk for physical and sexual abuse as children. This includes sexual abuse and other forms of interpersonal violence, which may predispose some gay men to have negative mental and physical health outcomes (Guarnero, 2001; Kalichman, Gore-Felton, Benotsch, Cage, & Rompa, 2004; Krahe, Scheinberger-Olwig, & Schutze, 2001; Sandfort, de Graaf, Bijl, & Schnabel, 2001). In a nonclinical sample of 942 homosexual and heterosexual adults, 46% of gay men reported a history of childhood same-sex molestation compared to 7% of their heterosexual counterparts (Tomeo, Templer, Anderson, & Kotler, 2001). In a study utilizing a probability sample of 2,881 urban gay men, 20% reported a history of childhood sexual abuse, primarily by non-family perpetrators (Paul, Catania, Pollack, & Stall, 2001). Niesen and Sandall (1990) conducted a chart review of 201 gay and lesbian chemically addicted inpatients and found that nearly 50% reported a history of sexual abuse in childhood. Jinich and colleagues (1998) explored the prevalence of childhood sexual abuse among a nonclinical sample of 1,941 gay and bisexual men and found that one-quarter reported a history of childhood sexual abuse.

The development of trauma-related symptoms in gay men may also be influenced by violence and oppression in the form of homophobia (Cassese, 2001; Dillon, 2001). Homophobia can result in a "hate crime" or more subtle forms of oppression and discrimination (Klinger, 1996). In a community sample of 445 young gay and bisexual males, Vives (2002) found that 75% experienced verbal harassment related to sexual orientation and 33% reported physical violence related to sexual orientation. Sexually abused in a cultural context that stigmatizes, devalues, and punishes homosexuality, gay men may thus present for treatment with complex forms of trauma-related disorders (King, 2001).

One reason for the risk of increased trauma among gay men is that as children they tend to display behaviors and attitudes frequently associated with gender atypical behavior. Brooks (2001) contended that gender atypical boys are at increased risk for sexual, physical, and emotional abuse. Violence is often used against these gender atypical boys to punish their "misbehavior" and to teach other boys the "rules" for socially acceptable male behavior. Males who behave in a gender atypical "feminine" manner are at high risk for being stigmatized, ostracized, and abused. Robertson (1997) further postulated that mental health professionals compound the difficulties some of these boys struggle with by diagnosing them with gender identity disorder in childhood. He contended this diagnosis often leads to treatment that is designed to "change" homosexuality in boys, which is of questionable value since 75% of such nontraditional boys are likely to be gay-identified later in life (Swidey, 2005). Additionally, there is an elevated risk of attempted suicide for younger gay men (and lesbians) that may also be attributed to a history of abuse (Fergusson, Horwood, & Beautrais, 1999; Gonsiorek, Sell, & Weinrich, 1995; Herrel et al., 1999; Vives, 2002).

As adults, gay men have an increased risk for anxiety and mood disorders, which are frequently associated with a history of trauma (Dillon, 2001; Edwards, 1996; Herrel et al., 1999; Levinson, 2000; Magel, 2002; Sandfort et al., 2001; Tillotson, 1997). Gay men also have greater than expected rates of chemical and substance abuse when compared to other men, which is also associated with physical and sexual abuse (Gonsiorek et al., 1995; Magel, 2002; Stall & Purcell, 2000).

One of the most disturbing outcomes of abuse in gay men is its relationship to high-risk sexual behavior and, consequently, HIV/AIDS. In a study of the impact of perceived coercion in sexual abuse for gay and bisexual Latino men, those who reported coercion also reported more alcohol use, more incidents of unprotected anal sex, and more sexual partners (Dolezal, 2002). Gay men, particularly gay men of color, are at high risk for HIV/AIDS and report greater then expected rates of childhood sexual abuse and other forms of trauma (Kalichman et al., 2004). Specifically, men who are abused are more likely to report engaging in high risk sexual behavior, including unprotected anal intercourse, compared to their nonabused counterparts (Jinich et al., 1998; Kalichman et al., 2004). Indeed, regardless of sexual orientation, coercive sexual experiences in childhood may be related to engaging in a wider array of sexual behaviors in adulthood (Stevenson, 2000), including high-risk behaviors for HIV.

Kalichman and colleagues (2004) found that childhood sexual abuse was associated with an increased risk of unprotected anal receptive intercourse, trading sex for money or drugs, self-report of having HIV, and nonsexual violence for a sample of gay and bisexual men. Jinich and colleagues (1998) found that gay and bisexual men who were abused were more likely to engage in unprotected anal sex compared to their nonabused counterparts in the preceding year. Perceptions of being coerced sexually as a child were also associated with a high incidence rate of adult HIV infection. Paul and colleagues (2001) also found that gay and bisexual men with a history of childhood sexual abuse reported higher risk sexual behavior than their nonabused counterparts. This high-risk sexual behavior was mediated by substance abuse, patterns of sexual contacts, and partner violence. The authors of the study suggested a history of childhood sexual abuse among men who have sex with men predisposes those with histories of such abuse to heightened patterns of sexual risk. Gonsiorek and colleagues (1995) posited that the explanation for negative behavioral health outcomes for gay men is that, although homosexuality is not associated with psychopathology, stressors in the lives of gay men, including a history of physical and sexual abuse, may result in a greater incidence of trauma-related symptoms, including high risk sexual behavior.

GAY IDENTITY DEVELOPMENT

As previously noted, the result of childhood sexual abuse frequently leads to distrust, shame, guilt, inferiority, confusion, isolation, and despair. This is particularly challenging for young gay men trying to reconcile an affirmative gay identity in a culture that largely disdains homosexuality despite increasing evidence that sexual orientation begins in the womb (Swidey, 2005). In the 1970s, investigators began to examine the complex socialization process known as "coming out" in a series of descriptive studies of gay men, which provided an important framework for research on the psychological well-being of gay men (Dank, 1971; Warren, 1974; Weinberg, 1970). These early descriptive studies led to the development of the most widely accepted description of the process of gay identity formation, the Homosexual Identity Formation Model (HIF; Cass, 1979). In the HIF model, Cass proposed that gay men and lesbians change from prehomosexual to homosexual by reconciling conflicts about being gay and moving through six stages of change. HIF is a dynamic process composed of self-identity, objective behavior, and others' perceptions that moves the individual from one stage of gay identity to the next. The six discrete stages of HIF are: (a) Identity Confusion, (b) Identity Comparison, (c) Identity Tolerance, (d) Identity Acceptance, (e) Identity Pride, and (f) Identity Synthesis. The first three stages concern the question "Who am I?" while the latter three stages concern the question "Where do I belong?"

In Stage 1 (Confusion), the individual experiences an unformed self-perception (or perhaps a presumption of heterosexuality), which includes behaviors, desires, and thoughts that may be labeled as "homosexual" and cause internal conflict. In addition, others' perceptions/desires for the person to choose heterosexuality increases confusion and discomfort. In Stage 2 (Comparison), the individual has the recognition of being "different"—that one's thoughts, feelings, and behaviors may be incongruent with societal and even familial expectations or assumptions. Stage 3 (Tolerance) reflects the growing recognition within the individual that he or she may be gay and also includes a great deal of ambivalence about being "different."

At Stage 4 (Acceptance), an individual enters into the "Where do I belong?" aspect of the HIF process. The individual begins to claim a personal identity as a gay person, which he or she may or may not disclose to others. The Acceptance Stage is a prerequisite for pursuing healthy adult intimate relationships, which developmental theorists characterize as the struggle for intimacy versus isolation (Erikson, 1997). Stage 5 (Pride) is characterized by a rebellion against being "closeted" and an identification (or perhaps overidentification) with all things "gay." Finally, Stage 6 (Synthesis) is a characterized by the integrated, nondefensive identity as a gay person. The individual is comfortable in his or her sexuality and identity.

It is imperative that clinicians working with gay clients understand and appreciate the HIF model and how this relates to the "coming out" experience in order to understand how sexual abuse may distort this developmental process. In the author's clinical experience, this impact of abuse, which frequently includes the trauma-related emotional states of shame, confusion, isolation, and despair, may retard this process and lead to a self-loathing and a self-defeating identity.

Clinicians treating gay men must also understand the complex impact of gender, sexual orientation, and sexual abuse on self-identity and the ability to have intimate relationships. The majority of gay men (and others) abused as children have been abused by men. Male children who have been abused by men (regardless of sexual orientation) are likely to struggle with the implications of abuse for the "self" as a male. They have to face questions such as, "What kind of man am I going to be?" "Will I become a perpetrator?"

In addition to self-identity, gay men (unlike their male heterosexual counterparts yet similar to heterosexual women) must also be able to establish and maintain healthy sexual and emotional relationships with other men. Gay men who are abused manifest frequent struggles with self-identity and intimacy that may include high risk sexual and drug use behavior. In adulthood, they may be both victim and victimizer in their interpersonal relationships. Wright (2001) refers to a "spiral of risk" where gay men engage in high-risk behavior to "belong" or to avoid abandonment, which has a negative impact on self-esteem and health. Given the high incidence of sexual and emotional violence many gay men have experienced as children, gay male victims of sexual violence may also choose abused partners (King, 2001). As a result, sex, love, and intimacy are difficult to manage in many gay male relationships

TREATMENT

Facilitating Gay Identity Formation

Any provider working with gay men should utilize a normative frame for gay identity development such as the HIF model. Each gay/bisexual client's stage of identity, with particular attention paid to those in early stages of identity formation, should be assessed. As previously noted, the Stages of HIF are a normative process for coming out. Clients who are in earlier stages of HIF are more likely to seek out "nongay" identified providers who they perceive as "less biased." As clients gain clarity about their sexual identity, they are more likely to seek out gay role models, including gay-identified providers. Gay therapists may be particularly important for newly identified gay or lesbian individuals. Developmentally mature gay clients are more likely to be indifferent to the sexual orientation of their providers once they are assured of therapist competence and comfort with gay individuals.

Clinicians need to educate gay clients about the coming out process and how this process may impact perceived well-being, recognizing that gay men with a history of abuse may have trouble meeting those challenges. Childhood sexual abuse and its associated shame for many gay men may easily translate to a "shameful" existence that includes substance abuse, unsafe sex, mood and anxiety disorders, underemployment, lack of intimacy, and loss of meaning in life. This developmental process is expected to be even more complicated for those gay men who were abused by clergy since the betrayal is of such a basic trust and, as noted earlier, can be akin to incest trauma.

When working with youthful clients, mental health providers need to be aware that many gay adolescents and youth are quite isolated. Many gay youth need positive gay role models who have meaningful work and relationships. Over the past several years, a number of support groups, religious organizations, Web sites, and other multimedia have been created to meet the needs of gay and lesbian individuals. These resources may also prove helpful to mental health professionals working with gay youth.

Treating Mental Health Disorders

Health providers should assess abuse histories, including CPSA, for all clients, including gay males. In addition to questions about physical and sexual abuse, assessments for gay and bisexual individuals should include questions about harassment related to gender atypical behavior in childhood and other forms of gay specific abuse/harassment. These include "gay bashing," "spiritual" interventions designed to change gay identity, and incidents of being rejected/ridiculed by others (parents/guardians, the military, church groups) as a result of being gay. Abuse and rejection themes, often with onsets at an early age, are central to the lives of many gay men and lesbians struggling with mental disorders and engaging in high-risk sexual and drug use behavior.

Many abused gay men present for treatment in emotional states closely linked to their trauma histories: distrust, shame, guilt, inferiority, confusion, isolation, and despair. Additionally, the results of trauma can be seen in low self-esteem, high rates of anxiety, depression, substance abuse, sexual risk taking, a lack of intimacy, suicidal behavior, and symptoms associated with post-traumatic stress disorder as well as character pathology including borderline personality disorder. Gay men who are abused by other males, including male clergy, may also be concerned that the abuse "made them gay." Clinicians need to be prepared to explore these concerns keeping in mind that current data does not support a relationship between sexual orientation and sexual abuse (Stevenson, 2000).

When working with gay men, initial assessments need to be modified to evaluate particular risk factors. Gay and bisexual young adults with histories of abuse are at increased risk for suicide and providers should assess this risk and intervene as needed. Gay men who have been sexually abused are also at increased risk for HIV/AIDS and other sexually transmitted diseases. Each gay and bisexual male client should receive a risk assessment for HIV/AIDS and primary and secondary prevention intervention as needed, including awareness of their HIV status and a referral for counseling and testing as needed. Particular attention should be paid to the relationship of abuse, substance use, and HIV risk behavior. A medication consult should be considered as part of the assessment process as the use of antidepressant and antianxiety medication is often important adjuncts to the treatment process.

The conditions for recovery in trauma victims, which Herman (1992) and others have described, can be modified and successfully utilized with traumatized gay men, including those abused by clergy. These conditions include: a healing therapeutic relationship, a focus on safety, a process of remembering and mourning the trauma, a reconnection with ordinary life, and a sense of commonality with others who may have been abused. Each of these phases and how they related to working with gay men will be discussed.

The Healing Relationship

The healing relationship facilitates working through a number of developmental challenges abused individuals confront. Erickson (1997) proposed that human beings are destined to struggle with basic trust and distrust, autonomy and shame, initiative and guilt, industry and inferiority, identity and confusion, intimacy and isolation, generativity and stagnation. Individuals traumatized as children frequently struggle more with these developmental challenges. In successful treatment, a client should experience empowerment and autonomy and take initiative, particularly concerning their abuse history. The healthy therapeutic relationship fosters a sense of internal locus of control and industriousness. For the gay client, it nurtures an affirmative gay identity, promotes intimacy with others, and facilitates existential questioning and meaning.

Safety

A significant challenge in working with traumatized individuals is their tendency to engage in unsafe behavior, including high-risk sexual and drug use behaviors as well as suicidal behaviors. Gay men engage in all of the risky behaviors observed in other survivors. They also engage in behavior that is more prominent among gay and bisexual men, including the use of "designer drugs" and having sexual encounters with anonymous partners. It is very difficult to build and maintain a healing relationship and facilitate developmental change until survivors are able to reduce their risky behavior. Depending on the risk and safety issues involved, clinicians should utilize contracts for safety (particularly for suicidal survivors), promote relaxation training and other self-soothing skills, and rely on motivational interviewing for substance using clients. For the gay client, mental health providers must be particularly aware of the risk of HIV infection associated with risky sexual behavior. HIV prevention interventions, which are both skill based and utilize techniques of motivational interviewing, should be utilized. Additionally, there are a number of cognitive behavioral techniques that may be used to treat sexually compulsive behavior that is a significant problem for some gay men. Finally, it should be remembered that the risk for suicidal behavior may be particularly acute for HIV–infected and traumatized gay men with a history of major opportunistic infections and cognitive impairment (Forstein, 1994).

Remembering and Mourning

The process of remembering and mourning traumatic life experiences can be accomplished only in the context of a healing relationship and relative safety. The choice to confront trauma rests with the survivor. Gay male survivors of childhood sexual abuse, including CPSA, present for treatment with all of the usual positive and negativex coping strategies survivors use to manage their traumatic past. There have been a number of empirically based cognitive behavioral interventions developed that have been designed to promote self-care, facilitate reclaiming traumatic memories, and assist survivors with managing the affect associated with these memories. Some interventions include confronting the abuser or utilizing other surrogate experiences that approximate this process of confrontation. These techniques all rely on what Herman (1992) refers to as the "action of telling a story." For gay men, this storytelling is character-ized by a search for narrative events that would explain their symptoms of trauma (Burnham, 1994).

In addition to remembering and mourning childhood sexual abuse, many gay men must also remember and mourn the loss of their childhood innocence, which was stolen as a result of abuse related to being a gender atypical child. Many others have also been subjected to sexuality-based abuse as adolescents and adults, including gay bashing and being ostra-cized from peer and family groups. Many of the techniques used to explore childhood sexual abuse can be easily adapted and used to explore the experience of being targeted as a gay youngster.

Reconnecting to the Self and Others: Making Meaning

McCann and Pearlman (1990) identified core needs that trauma survivors struggle with in their interactions with others: to be safe, to trust, to have some control, to feel self-worth, and to be close to others. Gay men with a history of sexual abuse frequently have problems in these areas of self-identity, connection, and commonality. Traumatized gay men who have been able to reconcile their trauma experiences move from "victim" to "survivor" and are able to tolerate painful feelings, counter self-blame, be alone without being lonely, self-soothe when distressed, anticipate the consequences of their actions, set and maintain appropriate boundaries with others, and enter into mutually supportive, give-and-take relation-ships (Rosenbloom & Williams, 2002). They do not abuse drugs, alcohol, and/or sex. Their life has purpose beyond their own pain and suffering.

Coming out as both gay and abused is often important for many gay survivors. Many gay men seek comfort and meaning in joining civic and fraternal organizations that support the gay community. Reconnecting to the spiritual is also an important component of recovery for many gay men. Unfortunately, the teachings of many religious denominations regarding gay people make reconnecting to their childhood faith difficult for many gay men. The institutional reinforcement of shame for being gay replicates the abuse experience for gay victims of CPSA. Nonetheless, many gay men with a history of CPSA report a spiritual void in their lives. Rather than return to a faith that condemns them, many join other denominations whose teachings affirm their life choices and sexuality.

The ability to form and maintain relationships is central to recovery. It cannot be overestimated how important the development of a network of family, friends, and colleagues are for recovery from abuse. Most gay men must develop a "constructed" rather than a biological family since most still do not have children. "Friends" often form the core of a constructed family. This is particularly true for gay men and others who may be alienated from their family of origin. Although most families manage their cognitive dissonance about homosexuality and are able to love and support their gay children, others reject them. Most gay men, like others, desire a primary intimate relationship. As has been widely noted elsewhere, intimate relationships are particularly fraught with anxiety and problems for traumatized individuals. Gay men with a trauma history are frequently challenged in developing and maintaining intimate relationships. Therapists must be able to facilitate the frequently bumpy ride many traumatized individuals confront in finding meaning through intimacy.

CASE STUDIES

The following two clinical examples provide an overview of the recommended treatment approaches discussed previously for working with abused gay men at different stages of gay identity development. The first case is of an older gay male who has never resolved a coherent sexual identity and was victimized by other children as a result of gender atypical behavior. The second case concerns a gay male with a clear identity, a history of CPSA, and multiple somatic complaints.

Case 1: Early Stage of HIF Treatment for a Traumatized Gay Men

PS is a 62-year-old married affluent male professional who has maintained a secret life of intermittent anonymous sexual encounters with men for the past 40 years. These anonymous encounters were, until recently, divorced from relationship and attachment (HIF Stage 1: Confusion). Some of his earlier memories included being "in love" with his male babysitter and being taunted as a "sissy boy" by his stepfather. He clearly was a gender atypical child. All of his sexual fantasies, beginning in early adolescence, focused on other boys/men. He also reported a history of coercive childhood sexual abuse by older neighborhood boys beginning at age 9 and ending at age 11.

PS's presenting problem in therapy was that for the first time in his life, he had become friendly and affectionate with one of his young male sexual partners and was afraid that his wife would discover his infidelity. He reported that he loved his wife as a "sister" but that he had never had a satisfactory intimate encounter with any female, including his wife. He described his feelings for this young man as "being in love for the first time in my life." When asked about his sexual orientation, PS winced, became flushed, looked over his shoulder, and whispered, "I might be gay but I try not to think about it." He reported a self-identity increasingly at odds with his self-perception, his current behavior, and his role as a perception of himself as a "married man." In short order, PS ended his friendship/ romance with this other man, abruptly left therapy, became depressed, was hospitalized, and treated with antidepressant medication. He returned to therapy some months later, overwhelmed with guilt, loneliness, and despair.

Upon his return, the focus of treatment was on the first three "Who am I?" stages of HIF rather than other external life changes PS might make in response to a more coherent identity. There were no easy answers for the dilemma that PS confronted, but relying on a developmental approach was helpful. Assisting this client with the question, "Who am I?" became the central focus of the initial phase of treatment. Much time was spent helping him to manage his anxiety and fear that if he were "truly gay" he would then need to leave his marriage. It can be quite helpful to counsel patients that first they need to know who they are and then they can decide whether to disclose this information to anyone else or make changes in the circumstances of their life. This patient needed to have an honest relationship with himself before he could address other issues. For many, it is also important to explore the meaning of sexual abuse and its relationship to sexual orientation since many gay men question if sexual abuse "made them gay."

Case 2: Later Stage Treatment for a Sexually Abused Gay Men

WA is a 48-year-old Black male who reported knowing he was gay from early childhood. He had had two long-term relationships with male partners in the past, although he now describes himself as "born again virgin." He was generally quite open about being gay although he had never disclosed his sexual orientation with his mother. He reported little ambivalence about leading a gay "lifestyle" (HIF Stage Four: Acceptance).

The patient was referred for mental health treatment after being diagnosed with a psychosomatic disorder by his primary care provider. The client had repeatedly sought emergency care for a host of physical complaints for which no acute illness could be identified. This increase in visits to the ER began after he was diagnosed with HIV disease two years previously. The client's health status was stable, his immune system largely intact, and he had no major opportunistic infections associated with HIV/AIDS. Given WA's relatively healthy immune system, it was highly unlikely he could have any of the infections for which he sought treatment. Indeed, most of WA's free time was spent "researching" HIV disease so that he was aware and could rationally articulate the futility of his ER visits. However, he would become anxious during unstructured times of the day and on weekends and then begin to ruminate about HIV/AIDS, which resulted in panic attacks and subsequent visits to emergency services.

Although the client had practiced safer sex consistently since his late 20s, he reported having had a "cocaine" problem in his early 20s, which led to frequent sexual partners and was likely when he became infected with HIV. He reported being gang raped at least once during a drug-induced state when he attempted to barter sex for drugs.

WA reported that from the ages of 10 to 12, a male clergy member associated with a chorus in which he participated repeatedly molested him. Soon after WA began to be molested, he developed a series of physical ailments (stomach aches, fatigue, nausea, diffuse pain) for which no cause was ever found. As a result, WA was identified as a "sickly child" and frequently kept home from school and choir practice by his mother. He reported that he was also "bullied" by other male children during this period of time and that being ill was a way to avoid this violence. Thus began a long history of somatic complaints whenever WA became anxious or depressed, which persisted to the time of his presentation for treatment. The diagnosis of HIV disease was the first time WA had what he referred to as "a serious disease" and his typical somatic response to stress was less tenable.

The thrust of early treatment for WA was to explore the relationship of childhood CPSA and the development of psychosomatic complaints. Although the link might seem apparent, WA was completely stunned to realize that his symptoms first appeared at almost the exact moment he began to be molested. Although, his symptoms did not magically disappear after this realization, they were significantly reduced after he acknowledged the link between childhood sexual abuse and somatic symptoms. He also benefited by learning stress management techniques to employ when he was feeling anxious or depressed as well as having a prescription for an antianxiety medication, which he could take as needed.

Although the primary focus of therapy was not on gay identity formation, the patient was troubled by not disclosing his sexual orientation and

HIV status to his mother. He was preoccupied with the thought that his mother had a "right to know" about his identity. Although WA described a warm and loving relationship with his mother, the fact that his orientation had never been acknowledged (and more recently his HIV status) had created a distance that he did not desire. At his initiative and with a great deal of therapist support, the client disclosed being gay and having HIV to his mother. She was relieved to finally have him acknowledge his homosexuality, which she had always suspected. Although very concerned about his HIV, she was relieved that he was in such good health. Interestingly, although WA did not disclose his childhood abuse to his mother, he did disclose his irrational fears of illness and engaged in an ongoing dialogue with her about his lifelong struggle with somatic complaints, which he found quite helpful.

WA never had any difficultly describing his abuse or expressing his disdain for his perpetrator, who had long ago "disappeared" from the congregation for unspecified "personal problems." Rather than confront the abuser, this client felt the need to confront his biological father who was the other man in his life who he felt betrayed him. For the first time, he forged a semblance of a relationship with his father.

Treatment also explored the patient's identity formation as a Black man. Although he had two intimate relationships with men, he had never dated or had an ongoing intimate relationship with another Black male. Initially, he indicated he had no idea why he preferred White male partners but gradually came to the realization that Black men represented the perpetrator to him since his perpetrator was Black. He also felt that unresolved issues related to his father contributed to his estrangement from Black men. WA described both fearing and desiring men of color. This was evident during his troubled past when he frequently sought out and engaged in high-risk drug and sexual behavior anonymously with Black men. In contrast, he perceived White men as generally safer, although he felt less erotically drawn and less culturally "in sync" with them, which resulted in "boredom" and contributed to his failed relationships. Over a period of time, WA began to seek out other men of color, including a support group of men with HIV. He soon began dating one these men.

CONCLUSION

Substantial evidence suggests gay men are at increased risk for a range of trauma experiences, including childhood sexual abuse, physical assault, and verbal harassment. In order to assist gay men who are abused, it is important to understand the developmental challenges they experience trying to reconcile an affirmative identity in the context of abuse. Mental health professionals should adopt a normative frame for gay identity development. The HIF Model discussed in this article provides such a framework. Efforts should be made to determine a gay/bisexual client's HIF stage of identity formation and interventions designed accordingly. Prior to beginning treatment, abuse histories should be taken for all gay clients, including questions about CPSA. In addition to questions about physical and sexual abuse, assessments for gay and bisexual individuals should include questions about harassment related to gender atypical behavior in childhood and other forms of gay specific abuse/harassment. Each gay and bisexual male client should also receive a risk assessment for HIV/AIDS and primary and secondary prevention intervention as needed. Upon completion of an initial assessment, trauma treatment protocols (Herman, 1992; Linehan, 1993) can be modified and successfully utilized with traumatized gay men.

There is also a need for clinicians, who are sensitive to the issues of gay identity development, to be engaged in prevention and advocacy designed to reduce the incidence of CPSA and to protect the needs of gender atypical boys. These efforts may include educating the clergy about sexual abuse as well as treating clergy who are at risk for abusing children and may have other mental health disorders. Prevention and advocacy efforts should also extend to working with guidance counselors, school psychologists, teachers, coaches, and others who work with youth and educating them about the needs and vulnerabilities of gender atypical boys.

There are almost no studies that specifically examine the incidence and impact of CPSA for gay men. Research is needed on how clergy abuse, as opposed to other forms of abuse, might impact sexual identity formation and mental, physical, and spiritual health in gay men. Furthermore, interventions should be developed and tested for treating gay men and others with a history of CPSA.

REFERENCES

Brooks, F. (2001). Beneath contempt: The mistreatment of non-traditional/gender atypical boys. In J. Cassese (Ed.), *Gay men and childhood sexual trauma: Integrating the shattered self* (pp. 1–17). Binghamton, NY: The Haworth Press.

Burnham, R. (1994). Trauma revisited: HIV and AIDS in gay male survivors of early sexual abuse. In S. Cadwell, R. Burnham, & M. Forstein (Eds.), *Therapists on the front line: Psychotherapy with gay men in the age of AIDS* (pp. 379–404). Washington, DC: American Psychiatric Association Press.

Cass, V. (1979). Homosexual identity formation: A theoretical model. *Journal of Homosexuality, 4*, 219–235.

Cassese, J. (2001). Introduction: Integrating the experience of childhood sexual trauma in gay men. In J. Cassese (Ed.), *Gay men and childhood sexual trauma: Integrating the shattered self* (pp. 1–17). Binghamton, NY: The Haworth Press.

Dank, B. (1971). Coming out in the gay world. *Psychiatry, 334*, 180–197.

Dillon, J. (2001). Internalized homophobia, attributions of blame and psychological distress among lesbians, gay and bisexual trauma victims. *Dissertation Abstracts International, 62*, (4-B).

Dolezal, C. (2002). Childhood sexual experiences and the perception of abuse among Latino men who have sex with men. *Journal of Sex Research, 39*, 165–173.

Doyle, T. (2003). Roman Catholic clericalism, religious duress, and clergy sexual abuse. *Pastoral Psychology, 51*, 189–231.

Edwards, L. (1996). Internalized homophobia in gay men: An investigation of clinical sensitivity among therapists. *Dissertation Abstracts International, 57*(6-B).

Erickson, E. (1997). *The life cycle completed: Extended version.* New York: W.W. Norton and Company.

Fergusson, D., Horwood, L., & Beautrais, A. (1999). Is sexual orientation related to mental health problems and suicidality in young people? *Archives of General Psychiatry, 56*, 876–880.

Fogler, J. M., Shipherd, J. C., Clarke, S., Jensen, J., & Rowe, E. (2008). Impact of clergy-perpetrated sexual abuse: The role of gender, development, and posttraumatic stress. *Journal of Child Sexual Abuse, 17*(3–4), 329–358.

Forstein, M. (1994). Suicidality and HIV in gay men. In S. Cadwell, R. Burnham, & M. Forstein (Eds.), *Therapists on the front line: Psychotherapy with gay men in the age of AIDS* (pp. 111–145). Washington, DC: The American Psychiatric Association Press.

Gonsiorek, J., Sell, R., & Weinrich, J. (1995). Definition and measurement of sexual orientation. *Suicide and Life Threatening Behavior, 25*(Suppl.), 40–51.

Guarnero, P. (2001). Shadows and whispers: Latino gay men living in multiple worlds. *Dissertation Abstracts International, 61*(11-B).

Herman, J. (1992). *Trauma and recovery.* New York: Basic Books.

Herrel, R., Goldberg, J., True, W., Ramakrishman, V., Lyons, M., Ostrow, D., et al. (1999). Sexual orientation and suicidality: A co-twin control study in adult men. *Archives of General Psychiatry, 56*, 867–874.

Jinich, S., Paul, J., Stall, R., Acree, M., Kegeles, S., Hoff, C., et al. (1998). Childhood sexual abuse in HIV risk taking behavior among gay and bisexual men. *AIDS and Behavior, 2*(1), 41–51.

Kalichman, S., Gore-Felton, C., Benotsch, E., Cage, M., & Rompa, D. (2004) Trauma symptoms, sexual behaviors and substance abuse: Correlates of childhood sexual abuse and HIV risk among men who have sex with men. *Journal of Child Sexual Abuse, 13*(1), 1–15.

King, N. (2001). Childhood sexual trauma in gay men: Social context and the imprinted arousal pattern. In J. Cassese (Ed.), *Gay men and childhood sexual trauma: Integrating the shattered self* (pp. 19–35). Binghamton, NY: The Haworth Press.

Klinger, R. (1996). Impact of violence, childhood sexual abuse, and domestic violence and abuse on lesbians, bisexuals and gay men. In R. Cabaj & T. Stein (Eds.), *Textbook of homosexuality and mental health* (pp. 801–818). Washington, DC: The American Psychiatric Association Press.

Krahe, B., Scheinberger-Olwig, R., & Schutze, S. (2001). Risk factors of sexual aggression and victimization among homosexual men. *Journal of Applied Social Psychology, 31,* 1385–1408.

Levinson, P. (2000). The relationship of gay related developmental stress to problems in living in college age men. *Dissertation Abstracts International, 61*(5-B).

Linehan, M. (1993). *Skills training manual for treating borderline personality disorder.* New York: Guilford Press.

Magel, N. (2002). Psychosocial predictors of health risk taking behaviors in gay men. *Dissertation Abstracts International, 63*(5-B), 2593.

McCann, I., & Pearlman, L. (1990). *Trauma and the adult survivor.* New York: Brunner/ Mazel.

Niesen, J., & Sandall, H. (1990). Alcohol and other drug abuse in a gay/lesbian population. *Journal of Psychology and Human Sexuality, 3,* 151–168.

Paul, J., Catania, J., Pollack, L., & Stall, R. (2001). Understanding childhood sexual abuse as a predictor of sexual risk taking among men who have sex with men: The urban men's health study. *Child Abuse and Neglect, 25,* 557–584.

Robertson, T. (1997) Gay male development: Hermeneutic and self psychological perspectives. *Dissertation Abstracts International, 57*(10-B), 6589.

Rosenbloom, D., & Williams, M. (2002). Life after trauma: Finding hope by challenging your beliefs and meeting your needs. In M. Williams & J. Sommer (Eds.), *Simple and complex post-traumatic stress disorder: Strategies for comprehensive treatment and clinical practice* (pp. 119–133) Binghamton, NY: The Haworth Press.

Sandfort, T., de Graaf, R., Bijl, R., & Schnabel, P. (2001). Same sex sexual behavior and psychiatric diagnoses: Findings from the Netherlands mental health survey and incidence study. *Archives of General Psychiatry, 58*(1), 85–91.

Stall, R., & Purcell, D. (2000). Intertwining epidemics: A review of research on substance use among men who have sex with men and its connection to the AIDS epidemic. *AIDS and Behavior, 4,* 181–192.

Stevenson, M. (2000). Public policy, homosexuality and the sexual coercion of children. *Journal of Psychology and Human Sexuality, 12*(4), 1–19.

Swidey, N. (2005, August 14). Gay? The evidence builds for how sexual orientation begins in the womb. *Boston Globe Magazine,* pp. 33–37.

Tillotson, D. (1997). Self-esteem and mood as predictors of sexual compulsivity in gay men. *Dissertation Abstracts International, 58*(5-B).

Tomeo, M.., Templer, D., Anderson, S., & Kotler, D. (2001) Comparative data of childhood and adolescence molestation in heterosexual and homosexual persons. *Archives of Sexual Behavior, 30,* 535–541.

Vives, A. (2002). The psychological sequellae of victimization based on sexual orientation: A structural equation model of predicting suicidality among lesbian and gay young adults. *Dissertation Abstracts International, 62*(12-B).

Warren, C. (1974). *Identity and community in the gay world.* New York: John Wiley and Sons.

Weinberg, M. (1970). Homosexual samples: Differences and similarities. *Journal of Sex Research, 6,* 312–325.

Wright, D. (2001). Illusions of intimacy. In J. Cassese (Ed.), *Gay men and childhood sexual trauma: Integrating the shattered self* (pp. 117–126). Binghamton, NY: Haworth Press.

Restorative Mediation: The Application of Restorative Justice Practice and Philosophy to Clergy Sexual Abuse Cases

Douglas E. Noll
Linda Harvey

The law and legal process involved in clergy-perpetrated sexual abuse (CPSA) is complex because it involves secular and religious authority. Because of its adversarial nature, legal processes may reinjure and traumatize victim-survivors, offenders, parishes, the church, and the community without providing a personal sense of justice or adequate reparation. Restorative justice offers processes that are respectful, nonadversarial, creative, and, most important, fair to all.

In this paper, we look at the law's response to CPSA cases in the Catholic Church. We choose the hierarchal Catholic Church because the problems within it have surfaced first and have been highly publicized. Nonetheless, it should be remembered that CPSA exists in all faiths and religious traditions, and it seems only a matter of time before attention is turned away from the Catholics to other faiths and traditions.

We begin with a brief history and overview of restorative justice, comparing criminal and civil justice processes to restorative justice. We will then briefly examine the scope of the problem of abuse in the Catholic Church by looking at the statistical information on criminal and civil cases. This will include a summary of civil settlements in the past five years in various dioceses. We consider the advantages and disadvantages of the criminal and civil responses to CPSA and propose how a restorative justice response could provide opportunities for healing, reconciliation, and settlement of difficult lawsuits not available under the criminal or civil system. We will propose what the attributes of a restorative justice mediation process should look like and present a case study comparing civil, criminal, and restorative justice approaches.

RESTORATIVE JUSTICE OVERVIEW

The History of Restorative Justice

Modern restorative justice began in 1974. Mark Yantzi, a young, full-time probation officer attached to the court in Kitchener, Ontario, encountered a case that intrigued him. Two young men had gone on a rampage in the town of Elmira, Ontario, slashing tires, breaking windows, and generally destroying everything in their path. They were captured and charged with 22 counts of property damage and vandalism. Yantzi was assigned the job of preparing the presentencing report for the court. One evening at a meeting with church volunteers, Yantzi casually asked, "Wouldn't it be interesting for these guys to meet with their victims?" The group's response was strong and unanimous: "Yes, arrange for the young men to meet their victims!" (Yantzi, 1998, p. 52). Despite Yantzi's deep reservations, he and David Worth, one of the church volunteers, met with the judge to talk about the idea. To their amazement, the judge agreed. Yantzi and Worth then met with the offenders, who agreed to the idea as well. The four retraced the evening and introduced themselves to the affected people at their front doors. The young men took notes about the damages they caused and moved on. After the two earned the money to pay for the damages, they, with Yantzi and Worth, went out on the path again. This time, they handed each household a check to repair the damage. Thus, the Victim-Offender Reconciliation Program (VORP) began in Canada.

Through Yantzi's Mennonite Church, the concept spread to Elkhart, Indiana, in the United States and a VORP program started there. A few years later, the idea moved to Fresno, California, through the efforts of Ron and Roxanne Claassen, and VORP was established on the west coast. From Kitchener, Elkhart, Fresno, and the Mennonite community in general, restorative justice began to grow internationally at a grassroots level.

The movement and philosophy of VORP did not receive attention from scholars and academics until the 1980s. The first use of the term *restorative justice* was in a paper by Howard Zehr (1985). Zehr looked at the problem of state justice, community justice, and covenant justice. He concluded:

> The central focus of the old paradigm is on the past, on blame-fixing. While the new paradigm would encourage responsibility for past behavior, its focus would be on the future, on problem-solving, on the obligations created by the offence. Restoration, making things right, would replace the imposition of pain as the expected outcome in new

paradigm justice. Restitution would be common, not exceptional. Instead of committing one social injury in response to another, a restorative paradigm would focus on healing. Retributive justice defines justice the Roman way, as right rules, measuring justice by the intention and the process. Restorative justice would define justice the Hebrew way, as right relationships measured by the outcome. (p. 80)

Zehr followed this paper with his groundbreaking book *Changing Lenses* (1990), which was the first extended discussion of the philosophy of restorative justice. Since then, more than a thousand journal articles and dozens of books have developed the theoretical aspects of restorative justice. At its core, however, restorative justice is based in practice, not in academic theory. To understand restorative justice generally, and its role in CPSA cases, one must grasp the essential differences between three justice models: the criminal law model, the civil law model, and the restorative justice model.

The Criminal Law Model of Justice

In simplified form, criminal procedure includes three components. First, a crime occurs and the offender is arrested. Second, a trial occurs and the offender is acquitted or found guilty. Then, finally, the offender is punished by imprisonment or death. At the conclusion of the process, justice is presumed done. There are a number of assumptions that come into play that are not always well considered when society defines behavior as a crime.

The focus of governmental attention is on the harmful act and the perpetrator. The dispute is not between the victim and the offender but between the state and offender. The state initiates a criminal action against the accused on behalf of society. The state has the exclusive power whether to charge a crime, what to charge, whether to continue the prosecution, whether to settle by plea bargain or try the case, and to decide what punishment to request from the court.

The offender is generally not allowed to tell his or her story and, to invoke constitutional rights, must repeatedly deny all responsibility and accountability for the wrong. Therefore, the offender is generally a passive, silent observer to the process. Likewise, the victim is not a participant in the system except as a witness. In many trials, the victim is excluded from the courtroom if he or she is to take the witness stand. The needs of the victim, offender, and community are largely irrelevant in a criminal prosecution. The prosecutor is primarily interested in obtaining a conviction and is not usually concerned with the broader social needs created by the offense. If the prosecution is successful, the offender is punished by fine, imprisonment, or death. The victim's multiple needs for justice (primarily vindication and validation) are assumed to be met by state-inflicted punishment.

Great social stigma is attached to criminal convictions and offenders suffer a severe loss of moral reputation. This loss persists long after punishment has been carried out and is, in effect, a further social punishment. Because of the severely harmful effects of conviction, the state is held to a very high standard of proof and strict procedural protections are theoretically in place to prevent wrongful conviction and punishment.

In summary, the focus is on the offender, the offense, and the punishment. In criminal law theory, minimal concern is given to the victim. Because of this, victims' rights groups, victim advocates, and other ad hoc victim programs have been implemented with varying degrees of success. The fact remains that a criminal prosecution is, by design, not oriented to the needs of the victim. Instead, prosecution is focused on assessing blame and punishment of the offender. Furthermore, criminal law focuses on the past, not the present or the future. One of the major weaknesses of criminal law theory is what to do with the offender when he or she is released from punishment.

The criminal response to the sexual abuse of children by clergy in the Catholic Church has not been robust. This is due in part to child victims of CPSA often not coming forward until they are adults, and the criminal prosecutions of CPSA being rare. Of the 4,392 priests accused of abusing children between 1950 and 2002, only 226 were criminally charged. Of those, 138 were convicted (John Jay College of Criminal Justice, 2004).

The Civil Law Model of Justice

When society defines behavior as a civil wrong (called a tort), a different set of assumptions come into play. The focus of attention is on the harmful act and the damage or loss caused by it. Unlike a criminal action, the act is construed as a private injury inflicted by one person on another. In simplified terms, the injured party (the plaintiff) initiates legal action against the offender (the defendant), controls the process, and has the power to settle, try, or dismiss the matter. If the injured party is successful, the court may award a judgment for damages payable by the offender, issue a coercive order such as an injunction, or declare rights between the parties. Civil remedies are therefore limited to a judgment for money, coercive orders, or declaratory judgments. While the offender cannot be imprisoned, the offender may be liable for substantial damages in serious cases. Often the offender is insured and the insurance company takes the burden of defending the offender and paying any judgment. Thus, when the offender is insured, the offender does not have to assume personal or financial responsibility for the injury.

Similar to criminal cases, the greater needs of the victim, offender, and community are largely irrelevant to a civil case except insofar as they help to prove damages. Likewise, the nature of cross-examination can subject victims and offenders to embarrassment, indignity, and disrespect. In contrast to criminal cases, society assumes that monetary compensation, rather than punishment, equals justice. Because the harm attached to civil liability is considered less than that of criminal liability, the procedural safeguards are much more relaxed. The burden of proof is much lower, the evidentiary standards are not as strict, and the mode of trial is not as tightly controlled. In addition, most civil cases are settled out of court before trial by negotiation. This settlement process is encouraged by the courts. Finally, the tax consequences to the victim can be significant in nonphysical injury cases if a substantial payment is received from the offender or the offender's insurance company.

In CPSA cases, civil lawsuits against the Catholic Church have been far more common, and the larger settlements have been nationally publicized. According to the John Jay College of Criminal Justice (2004) study, reported CPSA–related costs totaled $573 million, with $219 million covered by insurance companies. The study noted that the total dollar figure was much higher than reported, because 14% of the dioceses and religious communities did not provide financial data. In addition, the reported costs did not include settlements made after 2002, including: Diocese of Orange, California, 2004, $100 million for 90 abuse claims; Diocese of Covington, Kentucky, 2006, up to $85 million for 361 people; Archdiocese of Boston, 2003, $85 million for 552 claims; Diocese of Oakland, California, 2005, $56 million to 56 people; Archdiocese of Louisville, Kentucky, 2003, $25.7 million to 243 victims; Diocese of Tucson, Arizona, 2005, a settlement trust worth about $22 million for more than 50 victims as part of a plan to emerge from bankruptcy protection; Diocese of Providence, Rhode Island, 2002, $13.5 million to settle 36 claims; and Diocese of Los Angeles, California, 2007, $660 million to settle 550 claims. In addition to the Tucson diocese, other dioceses have filed for bankruptcy protection, including the Portland, Spokane, Davenport, and San Diego dioceses (Zoll, 2005).

Not surprisingly, many victim-survivors have been extraordinarily dissatisfied with the results of the traditional justice system. In a 2004 *Washington Post* article (Finer, 2004), victim attorney Mitchell Garabedian, who participated in the negotiation of the Boston settlement, said, "It's not uncommon for victims to feel pain after a settlement because the validation . . . does not fill the emotional and spiritual void" (p. A3). Many victims are not finding justice in the court room, and the Catholic Church and its insurers are paying hundreds of millions of dollars in legal defense costs and settlements.

The Restorative Justice Model of Justice

The restorative justice model brings a third set of assumptions into play. The focus of attention is on the harmful act, the offender, the victim, and the community. The victim is an active, key participant in the process. The behavior is not just a crime or a civil wrong but is an injury to relationships within the community. Thus, unlike criminal and civil cases, the offense and injury is placed in a larger social context. The outcome of the restorative process, representing the wishes of the victim, the offender, and the community, should be granted great deference by the state authorities. In contrast, the victim and offender's desires would be irrelevant in a criminal prosecution and to a lesser degree in a civil lawsuit.

Restorative justice is a problem-solving approach to serious offenses involving the offender, the victim, and the community. It has been described as a philosophy, a practice, and an ideal. In general, a practice is considered restorative when (a) the parties are able to meet and talk about their experiences of the wrong; (b) the parties discuss and agree on how to make things as right as possible between them, recognizing that many wrongs are unrightable; and (c) the parties discuss and agree on how future safety might be assured. Thus, restorative justice practices make room for the parties to participate directly in the resolution of the harm caused by the offense. In contrast to criminal justice, restorative justice also sees crime in a larger social context, takes a problem-solving, forward-looking orientation, and encourages creativity and flexibility.

We can say that a process is more or less restorative depending on how many of these elements are present. This process definition permits wide latitude in actual practices, from integrative mediation to peace circles to family group conferences. The restorative degree of a practice or process can be measured by simply asking and answering whether and to what degree the elements of restorative justice are present.

A Comparative Analysis of Processes

The following hypothetical case illustrates the differences between the criminal, civil, and restorative responses to CPSA of juveniles. Father

Charles, a Catholic priest, sexually molested children under his care as pastor of a small parish. One of those children, Robert, is now an adult and has come forward with accounts of the abuse. How would the criminal, civil, and restorative processes differ?

In the criminal process, someone would make a complaint to the local police or sheriff. A report would be forwarded to the district attorney or local prosecutor for review and decision. If the prosecutor decided a crime had been committed and could be proved beyond a reasonable doubt, a criminal complaint would be filed, Fr. Charles would be arrested, and criminal proceedings initiated. Throughout this process, Fr. Charles would be represented by a criminal defense lawyer. Fr. Charles would be instructed by his lawyer not to talk to anyone. He would appear in court, and in most cases would not take the witness stand or say anything to the victim, the parishioners, or his superiors. His lawyer would often use techniques to discredit the victim on the witness stand, humiliating the victim if necessary through cross-examination. The result of the trial, if an acquittal, would set Fr. Charles free. Most likely, he would be forever tainted by the accusation. A conviction would send him to prison. The victim, Robert, would not obtain direct closure, but would have to be satisfied with a vicarious vindication through Fr. Charles's punishment.

In the civil process, Robert would hire an attorney to file a lawsuit against Fr. Charles and the archdiocese. The archdiocese would request that its insurance carriers defend it, and defense counsel would be appointed. Unlike the criminal case, the attorneys would be entitled to investigate each other's cases in pretrial discovery. At some point in the process, the case would be directed to civil mediation. At this mediation, Robert would be present with his attorney. In all likelihood, there would be archdiocese representatives present, but. Fr. Charles would not be present. In addition, insurance representatives would be on hand. Together, the archdicoese and its insurers would decide if the matter should settle and for how much. The mediator, a highly skilled attorney or retired judge, would discuss the strengths and weaknesses of the civil case with the lawyers and their clients in separate rooms. The conversations would concern negotiations over the amount of money to be paid to Robert by the insurance company. Robert's deeper needs for vindication and validation would not be discussed, and in most instances would be considered irrelevant by the professionals.

If the matter did not settle and went to trial, Fr. Charles probably would take the witness stand. He would be thoroughly cross-examined by the victim's lawyer. Likewise, Robert would be cross-examined by the archdiocese lawyer, who would do everything ethically possible to discredit the victim. If Robert won, it would be a verdict for money damages payable by Fr. Charles and the archdiocese. Typically, Robert's attorney would be paid approximately 40% of the total verdict and be reimbursed for costs. Whatever remained, if substantial, would be subject to income taxation, including the Alternative Minimum Tax. Under existing tax law, the possibility exists that Robert could end up paying more in taxes than actually received in the verdict. Assuming the victim collected the money, the matter would be considered closed.

A restorative justice process would be quite different from a criminal or civil proceeding. First, the archdiocese would have to receive a complaint of abuse. Ideally, the archdiocese would have a process in place for an independent authority to receive complaints and conduct impartial and neutral investigations. When notified of the complaint, the archdiocese would have to decide whether to engage in a restorative justice process. Explicit in this decision would be acceptance of accountability and responsibility to make things right with the victim-survivor if the claim seemed meritorious. At the time the complaint was lodged, an independent victim advocate would be appointed to assist Robert.

If the investigation determined that Robert's claim had some validity, the independent authority would advise the archdiocese and seek the archdiocese's consent to proceed. If the archdiocese refused to consent, the victim-survivor could pursue available legal remedies. If the archdiocese consented, the independent authority would contact trained restorative justice mediators to convene a restorative justice conference.

At the conference, Robert, the victim advocate, family members, Fr. Charles, leaders of the diocese, and perhaps representative parishioners would each share perspectives on the nature of the wrong and how it affected each person and the community. Robert would share his ideas on how to make things right, which might include financial compensation, counseling and therapy, education, and health care costs. The parties would discuss the scope and method of reparation until they reached agreement. Finally, the parties would talk about how to prevent this type of injury from occurring in the future. The agreement might include provisions for Fr. Charles to be assigned to duties not involving pastoral care, retirement, counseling, therapy, or anything else that the conference participants agreed would be useful. In addition, the archdiocese might agree to other prevention efforts, such as education of the lay and pastoral staff, more transparent processes for assignment of priests to parishes, more lay involvement in priest selection and assignments, etc.

If promises were made as part of the agreement, some form of accountability process would be decided on so that everyone understood the consequences of nonperformance. The agreement would constitute a binding contract that would require periodic reconvening of the conference to assess performance. Ultimately, the independent authority would monitor the progress of performance. Typically, agreements would call for performance of promises that might take years to complete. However, on successful completion of the agreements, the claim would be deemed closed.

The process would be modified in several respects if criminal or civil legal proceedings had been filed. In the criminal context, Fr. Charles would have to accept responsibility for a crimnal offense for restorative justice processes to work. If he was not willing to accept responsibility, the criminal process would take over. Upon acceptance of responsibility, the court could order the matter to the restorative justice conference. In addition to the matters identified above, the conference would discuss and recommend to the court how the criminal matter should be disposed. While the court would not be bound by the recommendation, in ideal circumstances the court would find the report and recommendation highly persuasive and influential. If the court did not accept the report and recommendation, the court would send the matter back to conference with directions.

If a civil lawsuit had been filed, the restorative justice conference would replace civil mediation or a judicially supervised settlement conference. The final agreement would include the usual settlement provisions included in civil settlements. The lawyers would attend the conference, but would not be the primary participants. Their role would be as advisors and counselors, not advocates.

In this hypothetical restorative justice process, one must be cognizant of the extreme power imbalance between the archdiocese and the victim-survivor. The power imbalance is always present just by the nature of the parties. Restorative justice deals with power imbalance through a requirement of voluntary agreement to participate, voluntary acceptance of responsibility for the wrong, and voluntary acceptance of accountability. Any party may withdraw from the process at any time for any or no reason whatsoever. As long as parties are engaged in the process, however, they are operating under an explicit agreement to collaborate and cooperate to make things as right as possible. This agreement renders the power imbalance found in coercive processes significantly less of an issue.

One might ask why the archdiocese would accept responsibility for the wrongs of one of its priests, rather than force the victim-survivor through the court system. The short answer is that very few, if any, CPSA cases have actually gone to trial. Since the vast majority haved settled before trial, it can be argued that a restorative process would be faster, less expensive, and more satisfying to everyone concerned. The experience in criminal restorative justice programs provides signficant empirical support for this outcome (e.g., see Evje & Cushman, 2000).

THE CATHOLIC CHURCH'S RESPONSE
TO CLERGY ABUSE

In response to the public outcry, the United States Conference of Catholic Bishops (USCCB) (2002) has invested much time and money to create some transparency around CPSA of children. The USCCB adopted a Charter for the Protection of Children and Young People in June 2002 at its semi-annual conference in Dallas. The charter created the National Review Board (NRB), a lay group composed of 11 distinguished individuals. The NRB was formed to oversee the creation and work of a new church office within the USCCB's quarters in Washington, DC. It is called the Office of Child and Youth Protection with a director and deputy director. The NRB commissioned two research studies from the John Jay College and also implemented audits of the 195 dioceses to see if they were complying with the new policies. Though the charter is a promise, each bishop responds individually in his diocese. In addition, an Ad Hoc Committee on Sexual Abuse was created within the USCCB in 1992, and is now permanently established as the Committee for Protection of Children and Young People of the USCCB. While these efforts are applaudable as correctives, they do not create a systemic restorative justice response to the problem of CPSA.

A RESTORATIVE JUSTICE MEDIATION MODEL
FOR CLERGY ABUSE CASES

CPSA is not only a violation of physical, psychological, and emotional well-being; it is also a violation of one's faith (see Guido, 2008). This makes reporting the abuse to the institution responsible for the harm very difficult. When the victim reports the abuse to the archdiocese and the claim is not turned into a criminal or civil lawsuit, the archdiocese has the power to believe the victim-survivor or not, to help or not, and to disclose what happened to the abusers or not. In the past when the victim-survivor was abused, the only recourse was to complain to the diocese. This usually resulted in pressure to remain silent "for the good of the Church" (Gavrielides & Coker, 2005).

One victim, initially abused at the age of 16 and whose initial reports were minimized by church hierarchy, spoke to the enduring effect of the abuse experience and the importance of a healing process, which restorative justice can be part of. He stated:

> To those who ask that we forgive and forget, please understand . . . the survivors, each of us in our own way, have spent our lives trying to move on, always weighing those two options. For some of us suicide, substance abuse, or violence ended the struggle early. . . . But we cannot escape the effects of the betrayals that were committed against us in God's name. They are inexorably woven into the texture of who we have become. That betrayal may not be a chargeable offense in a court of law. But there is no statue of limitation on its impact. And there should be no forgetting. (Investigative Staff of the Boston Globe, 2002, p. 9)

United Kingdom researchers Gavrielides and Coker believe that the Catholic Church has gone through two of three stages in the process of adopting a restorative justice model: denial and traditional justice. They suggest that the church is now ready for a third stage: restorative justice. They noted, however, that sexual abuse

> has a number of characteristics which made its handling by restorative justice or traditional justice processes very difficult. For example, investigating or prosecuting abuse carries an inherent danger of re-victimizing victims. The imbalance of power between the victim and offender is an intrinsic component of the victimization preventing victims from being able to exercise free choice. (Gavrielides & Coker, 2005, p. 14)

Therefore, they argue that these cases be handled by experienced mediators trained in restorative justice.

As we have discussed previously, restorative justice is a process that makes things as right as possible for the victim-survivor by addressing the moral accountability of the offender and the church through face-to-face dialogue. To distinguish it from other restorative justice practices and from traditional civil mediation, we call this process restorative mediation. We believe restorative mediation provides an opportunity to begin the process of emotional healing, gives personal peace for those involved, and assures future safety and security. Restorative mediation is a private, voluntary, informal, and party-controlled process where legal representatives or other supporting representatives may or may not be present, depending on the desires of the parties. We believe that restorative mediation is best facilitated by two mediators, both experienced in complex, emotional conflict management and in the specific problems attendant with sexual and other traumatic abuse.

The process begins with extensive preparation of the parties. Before the restorative mediation conference, the mediators meet separately with the parties and their representatives in confidential meetings. Much healing can occur for the victim and the offender if involved in these meetings. At the conference, the victim, the offender and/or religious representatives with authority, and community representatives come together to acknowledge the injustice and harm, to make things as right as possible, and to discuss the offender's future intentions.

In addition to its application in criminal and civil cases, restorative mediation can be used for current and past cases of clergy or religious sexual abuse where the victim seeks a restorative solution beyond what is available from legal process. It can be used for cases where the statute of limitations has expired; where there has been psychological or spiritual abuse, called "grooming," that did not result in an overt sexual act; for litigation that has been filed and resolved, but where further healing is needed; for cases where legal liability or sufficiency of evidence is in question; for cases where the surviving victim does not want to file a lawsuit; or for child sexual abuse and adult sexual boundary violations.

Restorative mediation is attractive to victims because they can experience a sense of justice not obtainable in the criminal or civil courts. The very act of confronting and conversing with church authorities and hearing them take responsibility for the wrong is sometimes all a victim seeks. Survivors of sexual abuse want the offender or offender's religious community to be accountable and remorseful. In addition, victims' seek assurance that others will not be harmed and there is appropriate treatment for the abuser. In some cases, compensation may be secondary and symbolic only to the degree of accountability and culpability accepted by the church. In other cases, victims want to be compensated for their treatment or other assistance for healing. Some want monetary compensation for their injuries. Monetary and nonmonetary outcomes can be handled in the same restorative mediation session.

In addition, some victim-survivors want to know the present location of the offender, if there are other victims, and if there have been life changes for the offender. Victim-survivors may also want the offender or offender's religious community to know firsthand the impact the abuse has had on their lives. Most of these needs or objectives will not be met in criminal or civil court action; all of these objectives are possible in a restorative mediation conference.

Victim Readiness

Not all victim-survivors are ready for the restorative mediation process. The mere thought of confronting the offender or church representatives in a private conference can be intimidating and may trigger emotional and psychological reactions. From our experience, restorative mediation should not be pursued until two to four years has elapsed from the last abuse encounter. Victim-survivors who are not in therapy of some type are encouraged to begin and those who are in therapy should consult with their therapist about readiness for the process.

Some victim-survivors may hold unrealistic views of the process and potential outcomes. For example, many victim-survivors think they can obtain millions of dollars as compensation. This expectation is created by publicity about lawsuits. The victim-survivor is most often not presented with the restorative justice option or other options for that matter. From the publicity, they may believe their only options are lawsuits or counseling. Part of the preparation for the conference involves deep reality testing to uncover what the true interests, needs, goals, and desires of the victim-survivor are. Victim readiness is indicated by completion of an investigation that acknowledges that a harm was done, and by a desire to heal, to have questions answered, to seek accountability from the church, to know the location and status of the offender, and to find peace through a nonadversarial process.

Role of Victim Advocate

Most dioceses have created a victim assistance coordinator or a victim's advocate. Sometimes, this has been a new position or expansion of an old position such as a Catholic Social Services counselor. These victim representatives work with victim-survivors reporting past child abuse to the diocese. They primarily represent the interests of the victim and advocate for their concerns and needs with diocesan authorities. A number of dioceses assist the victim-survivor with counseling and other needs before the claim is investigated. The keys to the success of a victim advocate sponsored by the dicoese are independence and confidentiality. The victim-advocate must be independent of influence by the diocese and must be able to maintain confidential communications with the victim-survivor.

Some victims are reluctant to contact victim assistance coordinators because they are perceived as being a part of the church that harmed them. In these situations, the victim-survivor may seek the assistance of an independent professional schooled in sexual abuse dynamics. This victim advocate is a companion and supporter throughout the process and is invited to be present during the restorative mediation conference.

Victim advocates must be trained in the psychology of traumatic relationships, understand the dynamics of post-traumatic stress disorder, have empathic communication skills, and be compassionate. Victim advocates must be knowledgeable about the criminal, civil, and restorative justice systems and must be able to draw on creative options to meet the needs of the victim-survivor.

Independent Investigation Determining Likelihood of Abuse

Victim-survivors have the right to an open and fair investigation of the facts without any pre-judgments or conclusions about the veracity of the complaint or the character of the offender. Unfortunately, many church investigations have been done in secrecy and confidentiality, betraying this basic right. Thus, the fairest process requires an independent investigator committed to involving the victim in the process.

The faith community (parish or congregation) where the offenses occurred also has a right to be informed of the allegations. The allegations should be stated objectively by a leader of the congregation or denomination. This right not only informs the community of the abuse, but allows other victim-survivors information that gives them the chance to come forward for help.

One of the most frustrating and painful experiences is an investigation that is slow or stalled. In a restorative process, Church institutions should provide a realistic time estimate for the investigation and should make periodic reports of progress. There are fewer obstacles to overcome when there is a Church-initiated restorative mediation following a complete, thorough, and independent investigation. Of course, this occurs when the Church is willing to be accountable and accept responsibility for making things as right as possible.

Acceptance of Responsibility

The investigation does not have to establish the veracity of the claim to a fault. Neither should the investigation establish responsibility sufficient to meet the legal requirements of a cause of action. Instead, the investigation should provide enough objective evidence for a reasonable person to conclude that, more likely than not, abuse occurred, regardless of when it occurred. The church should err on the side of the victim-survivor. If an independent investigation determines that the claim is not credible, the church should take steps to work with the parishioner in a positive way to minimize further estrangement. When responsibility has been established and accepted by the church, the restorative mediation process can move forward.

Preconference Meetings

One of the significant differences between restorative mediation and traditional legal mediation is the confidential preparation before the mediation conference. In this preparation process, the mediator works separately with the victim-survivor, the church representatives/offenders, and any other participants invited to the conference. The mediator constantly gauges the readiness of the individual parties for the conference. If the mediator determines that the conference will lead to further harm or revictimization, the mediator may decide to terminate the process.

The victim-survivor preparation includes the telling and sometimes retelling of the victim-survivor's story followed by an empathetic listening presence provided by the mediator. Trust, validation, and healing may occur during this preparation as the victim-survivor is perhaps truly heard for the first time by a compassionate and objective third person. In addition to storytelling, the victim-survivor is coached on the nature of the process, is asked to reflect on possible outcomes, and has the opportunity to ask questions of the mediator. The victim-survivor is asked to describe the effect the abuse has had on his or her life and to describe future hopes and plans and to discuss monetary and nonmonetary concerns. The mediator may recommend resources if the victim-survivor seeks further assistance.

In the preparatory meetings with church officials and representatives, the mediator must determine the degree of accountability and sincerity to make things right. The diocese or religious order must decide to be accountable for the wrong. Accountability will be expressed by an attitude of wanting to make things as right as possible with the victim, recognizing and acknowledging the nature of an unrightable wrong. Consistent with accountability, church authorities should be compassionate and sensitive to the victim's needs. A simple acknowledgment by a church representative of the devastation and harm suffered by the victim-survivor defuses anger, frustration, and the deep sense of betrayal. Church representatives should realize and be willing to acknowledge the effect of the harm on family members, spouses, children, and others in the broader community. The church should be willing to inform the public of the steps that have been taken to remove the offender from priestly or other church duties and disclose how many victims have been abused by a specific offender.

The Restorative Mediation Conference

Following the preparation process, the mediation conference is scheduled and a formal agreement to mediate is circulated to the parties for review and signature. Generally, the conference is convened at neutral, quiet location. The mediator normally meets separately with the religious representatives and the victim-survivor on the day of the mediation to answer any questions about the formal agreement to mediate, any legal mandates appropriate for the geographic location where the abuse occurred, conditions of confidentiality, and what has happened to the offender if he or she is not present.

After introductions at the conference, the mediator takes some time to describe the process and secure agreement on the ground rules and confidentiality agreements. The victim-survivor is invited to describe his or her experience of abuse, and church representatives are asked to summarize the victim-survivor's story. Each participant thereafter is invited to tell his or her story, with someone else summarizing back. When everyone agrees that the stories have been told and acknowledged, the discussion turns to making things as right as possible.

The victim-survivor is invited to talk about what interests, needs, goals, and desires should be met for healing to begin and for the victim-survivor to find the beginnings of peace. These needs vary, but may include apologies, compensation, counseling, health care, career preparation, parish educational forums, or assurances of future security. Many victim-survivors are traumatized because their faith has been stolen from them, and a conversation about faith and the possibility of its restoration usually is appropriate. The church representatives are invited to talk about their experience, to express remorse on behalf of the diocese, and to respond to the victim-survivor's needs. If the offender is present, forgiveness and reconciliation are not imposed, but at least apology occurs. At the end of the conference, which may last from four to eight hours, agreements are reduced to writing and initialed by the parties. Usually, the informal written agreements are converted to more formal legal agreements and later signed by the parties.

Follow-Up and Accountability

Once the mediation conference has been completed and appropriate agreements signed, the mediator may or may not accept the responsibility to monitor the postconference process to see that the agreements are kept. The independent or diocesan victim advocate may also monitor the implementation of agreements, or accountability management may be delegated to an independent agency. Generally, the mediator stays involved in the process until the agreements are fulfilled. Accountability management is a crucial part of the process. People tend to keep agreements when they know they are being watched. If challenges or difficulties arise during performance of the agreements, accountability management can provide for early and efficient interventions to bring the agreements back on course or make adjustments as needed.

OBSTACLES TO THE USE OF RESTORATIVE JUSTICE

Restorative mediation is not appropriate to determine the validity of an allegation. Likewise, the process is strictly voluntary and is not appropriate if there is any hint of coercion imposed on any person. Restorative mediation is not a shield to disclosure and is therefore inappropriate to keep the abuse a secret. Finally, restorative mediation is not appropriate if any party lacks a sincere desire to make things right or if there is doubt that the parties will carry out their agreements. Thus, if the church wishes to retain its power and control over the process, restorative mediation will not work.

There are obstacles to introducing restorative mediation into CPSA cases. First, many victims may have unrealistic expectations of what lawsuits will bring them. They naively believe that they will obtain justice in the courts through large monetary settlements or verdicts. Coupled with this is a strong desire for vengeance and retribution against the church. On the other side, many diocesan and religious order attorneys are advising their clients against restorative mediation because they are afraid if accountability is admitted, there will be exposure to further liability from other claimants. Many defense attorneys view CPSA through the lens of the traditional civil justice model and are not familiar with restorative justice. Many priest offenders are deceased or removed from ministry. Although some want to make amends, they are ignorant of or do not have access to restorative justice processes. Many church representatives and victim-survivors mistakenly think that restorative justice is about counseling or is about imposing forgiveness and reconciliation on the parties. Finally, many people in congregations want the problem to go away and simply do not want to invest the energy that is required by the restorative mediation process.

Other Situations

There have been instances where the victim wants a restorative mediation process but has not yet reported it to the religious body. Obviously, an investigation has not been done. The victim-survivor may contact a mediator to open a preliminary dialogue with the religious representatives. This conversation is informational and educational only. If the church representatives are interested and sincere in dealing with the potential claim restoratively, then the victim may feel more comfortable with the necessary reporting and other procedures.

Sometimes, the religious body has completed the investigation, proven the abuse, and wants to pursue a restorative process. A neutral and independent mediator may be retained to contact the victim to see if there is interest in pursuing this process. In some cases, the religious body may be contacted by a victim who has made allegations about an offender who has left the religious order or diocese. Again, a neutral and independent mediator may be retained to contact the alleged offender to first see if he will admit accountability and second, if he does admit accountability, would he be interested in a restorative process.

Regardless of whether a case ends in restorative mediation or not, the preparation can bring clarity to the victim or the offender/church representatives as to their options and choices for dealing with the claims. In many instances, the parties are empowered to make decisions and take control of their situation.

CONCLUSION

The power of restorative justice through the use of restorative mediation can aid the healing journey of victim-survivors, the church, offenders, and the larger community. While the process requires some initial vulnerability by all participants, the outcomes are generally superior to those provided in the criminal, civil, or canonical legal systems of justice.

The Restorative Justice Council on Sexual Misconduct in Faith Communities (RJC) is a national body of restorative justice practitioners, theologians, ministers, victim-survivors, and lawyers dedicated to bringing restorative mediation to bear on the problems of CPSA. More information about restorative mediation and other restorative justice processes of RJC can be found at its Web site: www.rjcouncil.org.

REFERENCES

Evje, A., & Cushman, R. C. (2000, May). A summary of the evaluations of six California victim offender reconciliation programs. Report to the California Legislature, submitted by the Judicial Council of California, Administrative Office of the Courts, Center for Familes, Children & the Courts. Retrieved June 11, 2008, from http://www.courtinfo.ca.gov/ programs/cfcc/pdffiles/vorp.pdf.

Finer, J. (2004, March 1). Settlement hasn't eased their pain: Payout to abuse victims leaves a void. *Washington Post,* p. A3.

Gavrielides, T., & Coker, D. (2005). Restoring faith: Resolving the Roman Catholic Church's sexual scandals through restorative justice. *Contemporary Justice Review, 18*(4), 345–365.

Guido, J. J. (2008). A unique betrayal: Clergy sexual abuse in the context of the Catholic religious tradition. *Journal of Child Sexual Abuse, 17*(3–4), 255–269.

Investigative Staff of the Boston Globe. (2002). *Betrayal: The crisis in the Catholic Church.* Boston: Little, Brown and Company.

The John Jay College of Criminal Justice. (2004, February 27). *The nature and scope of the problem of sexual abuse of minors by Catholic priests and deacons in the United States: A research study conducted by the John Jay College of Criminal Justice (National Clergy Sex Abuse Report).* Retrieved June 11, 2008, from http://www.usccb.org/nrb/johnjaystudy.

United States Conference of Catholic Bishops. (2002, June). *Charter for the protection of children and young people.* Retrieved March 31, 2006, from http:///www.usccb.org/ocyp/charter.shtml.

Yantzi, M. (1998). *Sexual offending and restoration.* Waterloo, Ontario: Herald Press.

Zehr, H. (1985). Retributive justice, restorative justice. Occasional paper no. 4. *New Perspectives on Crime and Justice Series, MCC Office on Crime and Justice.* Reprinted in G. Johnstone (Ed.), *A restorative justice reader* (pp. 69–82). Portland, OR: Willan Publishing.

Zehr, H. (1990). *Changing lenses* (1st ed., rev.). Scottdale, PA: Herald Press.

Zoll, R. (2005, June 9). Abuse costs for Catholic dioceses tops $1B. Associated Press. Retrieved September 11, 2008, from http://www.highbeam.com/doc/IPI-1091812599.htm

Problem and Solution: The Spiritual Dimension of Clergy Sexual Abuse and its Impact on Survivors

Kenneth I. Pargament
Nichole A. Murray-Swank
Annette Mahoney

Where we find trauma, we often find spirituality. Empirical studies have shown that many people seek support from their faith when they face crises in living, and from 50% to 85% of various groups find their spirituality helpful in the coping process (Pargament, 1997). This point holds true for survivors of sexual abuse. Many survivors describe the support they find from their spirituality. As one survivor of sexual assault put it, "I know who I am on a very deep, spiritual level, so I know nothing can destroy me" (Valentine & Feinauer, 1993, p. 220).

Even though expressions of spirituality are generally tied to health and well-being (see Koenig, McCullough, & Larson, 2001), there are times when spirituality becomes a part of the problem rather than a part of the solution. After all, life traumas impact people spiritually as well as psychologically, socially, and physically. This is clearly the case when it comes to clergy-perpetrated sexual abuse (CPSA). It is not hard to find anecdotal accounts of the powerful negative spiritual effects of CPSA on the individual's relationship with the church and God. One survivor commented, "I don't think I'll ever step foot in a church again . . . I lost my religion, faith, and ability to trust adults and institutions" (Matchan, 1992, p. 8). Another remarked, "God did not protect me either. Why would God not protect a helpless little boy? It was not fair. . . . Instead of welcoming and embracing [Jesus] as I want to, I really would like to knock him down. I am mad at him and his Father" (Anonymous, 1990, p. 119). More systematic research in this area is limited, but initial studies are consistent with these anecdotal comments: CPSA is often associated with a conflicted or broken relationship with God, a loss of trust in religious institutions, and an impaired ability to develop spiritually (e.g., Chibnall, Wolf, & Duckro, 1998; McLaughlin, 1994; Rosetti, 1995). These signs of spiritual distress have to be taken seriously; they have been linked empirically to increases in anxiety and depression, a loss of independent functional status, and a greater risk of mortality (e.g., Exline, Yali, & Lobel, 1999; Fitchett, Rybarczyk, DeMarco, & Nicholas, 1999; Pargament, Koenig, Tarakeshwar, & Hahn, 2001).

What then is the relationship between spirituality and trauma? There is no clear answer to this seemingly straightforward question. Unfortunately, social scientists and health professionals have largely ignored the spiritual dimension of trauma and, as a result, our understanding of the interface between these two domains is limited. Clearly, more research is needed in this area. But perhaps even more critical is the need for a way to *think about* spirituality in the context of trauma. In this paper, we offer a way to understand spirituality that may help to clarify the spiritual dimensions of one particular trauma, CPSA. We will suggest that spirituality can be a part of the solution to life crises, and it can be a part of the problem itself. Building on this conceptual foundation, we then consider some of the ways in which spirituality can be integrated more fully into our efforts to help survivors of CPSA.

SPIRITUALITY AS A SEARCH FOR THE SACRED

Many people think of "spirituality" in terms of a particular set of beliefs, practices, or experiences. Popular though it may be, this view is misleading, for spirituality is not a fixed or static institution; it is instead a process, one directly involved in our efforts to seek a particular kind of significance in life. Spirituality is "a search for the sacred" (Pargament, 1999, p. 12). Social scientists from Freud to Durkheim have noted that religion can serve a variety of functions, such as anxiety-reduction and the fostering of intimacy with others, identity, meaning and purpose, and self-development. Certainly, religion can play important psychological and social roles, but the most basic function of religion is spiritual. It is directed to the sacred. By sacred, we are referring not only to conceptions of God, higher powers, and divinity, but also to other aspects of life that take on spiritual character and significance by virtue of their association with the divine (Pargament & Mahoney, 2002). The sacred is the most central, motivating force that lies behind religion. As Paul Johnson (1959) once wrote, "It is the ultimate Thou whom the religious person seeks most of all" (p. 70). We can find evidence of spiritual motivation even at an early age. Consider the words of this nine-year-old boy:

> I'd like to find God! But He wouldn't just be there, waiting for some spaceship to land! He's not a person, you know! He's a spirit. He's like the fog and the mist. Maybe He's like something—something we've never seen here. So how can we know? You can't imagine Him, because He's so different—you've never seen anything like Him . . . I should remember that God is God, and we're us. I guess I'm trying to get from me, from us, to Him with my ideas when I'm looking up at the sky! (Coles, 1990, pp. 141–142)

FIGURE 1. The Search for the Sacred.

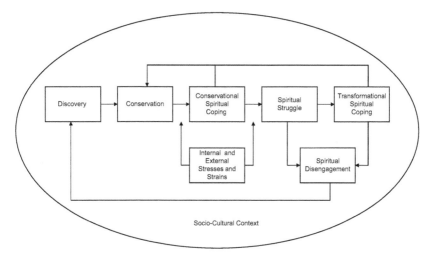

While religion serves multiple psychological and social functions, spirituality focuses directly on the search for the sacred (Pargament, 1999). By search, we are referring to three important dynamic and interrelated processes: the process of discovery of the sacred, the process of conserving or sustaining a relationship with the sacred once it has been found, and the process of transformation in the character or place of the sacred in the person's life as a result of internal or external stressors (see Figure 1 from Pargament, 2007). We elaborate on these three processes and their expression in the context of CPSA.

DISCOVERY

Psychologists have suggested that people's beliefs about the sacred grow out of several forces, including genetic factors (e.g., Bouchard, Lykken, McGue, Segal, & Tellegen, 1990), the child's intrapsychic capacity to symbolize and fantasize super-human beings (Rizzuto, 1979), and critical life events and challenges that reveal human limitations (Johnson, 1959). Of particular importance in shaping the child's understanding of the divine is the social context of family, institution, and culture (Kaufman, 1981). It is no accident that Christian children come to believe in Jesus, while Hindu children experience God through multiple divine entities, and Jewish children believe in the oneness of God. Of course, from a spiritual perspective these explanations are incomplete, for they neglect the "reality" of direct encounters with the divine, in which God essentially reveals God's self to the individual. Nevertheless, direct, empirical demonstrations of the "reality" of divine encounters take us beyond the scope of psychology. After all, we have no tools to measure God. However, we can use scientific methods to assess the varied ways in which people understand and experience the sacred.

Through religious institutions, culture, and personal experience, people learn to imbue many aspects of life with divine qualities, such as transcendence, ultimacy, and boundlessness (Pargament & Mahoney, 2005). The sacred can be discovered in the ordinary as well as in the extraordinary. As Durkheim (1915) wrote: "By sacred things one must not understand simply those personal beings which are called gods or spirits; a rock, a tree, a pebble, a piece of wood, a house, in a word anything can be sacred" (p. 52). Sacred objects include: time and space (the Sabbath, churches); events and transitions (birth, death); materials (wine, crucifix); cultural products (music, literature); psychological attributes (self, meaning); social attributes (compassion, community); and roles (marriage, parenting, work). People too can be sanctified. For example, one Roman Catholic young man said, "We were brought up that the priests . . . were the next thing to God on earth" (Matchan, 1992, p. 8).

There is nothing trivial about the sacred. Sacred matters matter. Empirical studies have pointed to several important consequences of the discovery of the sacred in a person's life (Pargament & Mahoney, 2005). First, the sacred elicits spiritual emotions. In some ways, we can think of sacred objects as love objects, for they can trigger feelings of adoration, gratitude, and uplift. They can also elicit feelings of awe as well as emotions of fear and humility. For many people, these emotional experiences become deeply embedded in memory throughout the lifespan. Second, the sacred becomes an organizing force, a superordinate goal or striving that lends coherence and direction to life (Emmons, 1999). Third, once discovered, the sacred becomes a resource people can draw on for strength, support, meaning, and satisfaction.

How does CPSA affect the process of spiritual discovery? Because most people discover the sacred as children, CPSA during this critical period is likely to have particularly devastating consequences for the normal development of spirituality. How, after all, can children develop a sense of faith and trust in religious leaders who have betrayed them? How can they develop any confidence in their teachings? How can they experience spiritual emotions, draw on their spirituality as a resource, or organize their lives around sacred objects so closely linked to pain and suffering? Many children, if not most, may not. Researchers have begun to describe the profound and long-lasting impact of CPSA on the child's relationship with God and the church (e.g., Fater & Mullaney, 2000).

CONSERVATION

Once discovered, people try to build and maintain a relationship with the sacred. After all, the sacred is precious. Religious institutions play an important role in this conservational process by encouraging people to follow a number of spiritual pathways: the pathway of spiritual knowledge (e.g., religious education, Bible study), the pathway of spiritual practice (e.g., ritual, virtuous actions), the pathway of spiritual relationships (e.g., church involvement, holy matrimony), and the pathway of spiritual experience (e.g., meditation, prayer; Pargament, 2007). Each of these paths is designed to sustain and strengthen the individual's relationship with the sacred. Prayer, for instance, can be understood as a way to "practice the presence of God" (cf. Brother Lawrence, 1975). Rituals represent concrete ways to create holy time and space in which people can regularly encounter the sacred.

Of course, most people encounter external life stressors or internal developmental changes over the course of their lives that threaten, damage, or violate the sacred. Even so, spirituality is quite resilient to these stressors, for people go to great lengths to preserve and protect their sacred values. Toward this end, they can take another spiritual pathway— the pathway of spiritual coping. People can draw on many methods of spiritual coping to conserve the sacred in times of stress. They can reframe negative events from a benevolent spiritual perspective. They can seek out spiritual support from God, clergy, and congregation members. They can engage in rituals of purification to regain their sense of spiritual direction. Empirical studies have shown that methods of spiritual coping such as these are often successful in helping people attain valued psychological, social, and spiritual ends (Ano & Vasconcelles, 2005; Pargament, 1997).

CPSA, however, puts a severe strain on the ability of the individual to conserve the sacred. Because the sacred has to do with one's deepest values, because the sacred elicits such powerful emotions, because the sacred is an organizing force, because people build relationships with the sacred, the violation of the sacred is an event that may shatter the individual's world. Mahoney and colleagues (2002) conducted a study that addresses this point. Following the September 11 attacks, they surveyed students in Ohio and in New York City about their perceptions of and reactions to the attacks. Many of the students reported that important spiritual values had been desecrated by the violence. Furthermore, those who perceived the attacks as a desecration (a violation of the sacred) reported more depression, anxiety, PTSD, grief, and were more willing to engage in extremist responses, such as the use of nuclear bombs and biological weapons on the countries sheltering the terrorists. These findings were replicated in another study of community residents who reported other types of desecration (Pargament, Magyar, Benore, & Mahoney, 2005). Perceptions of desecration, it appears, can elicit powerful social and emotional reactions.

CPSA is particularly destructive because it is a desecration on many levels. First, it is a violation of the most sensitive parts of the individual's identity, the soul, or that which makes the person uniquely human. As one survivor of CPSA wrote:

> This guy had my soul in his hand. It was devastating to know that someone would step out of the powers of spiritual liberty to take over someone else's soul . . . I still have anger about a lot of that and I think more of the anger is about the spiritual loss than anything to do with the sexual abuse. (Fater & Mullaney, 2000, p. 290)

Second, CPSA is a violation of a sacred role and relationship, one that has been set apart from others. Perhaps for this reason, sexual abuse perpetrated by fathers and father figures has been linked to greater trauma than abuse committed by other perpetrators (e.g., Browne & Finkelhor, 1986). In fact, it could be argued that sexual violation by clergy members represents an even greater desecration than violation by a biological parent, for clergy take formal vows to protect and nurture the spiritual well-being of all of their followers; they are legitimated to enact the role of God. Thus, when a clerical figure violates his or her ordination, responsibility, and privilege as a representative of God in a human relationship, it is as if God himself has committed the violation. Third, it is a violation of a sacred institution that legitimated the cleric, possibly cloaking the acts of the perpetrator and failing to come to the aid of the survivor. Fourth, CPSA is a violation of a set of rituals and symbols that were intertwined with the offending clergy and institutions. For example, one woman who had been abused by her minister at the age of 14 described her alienation from the rituals of her church:

"I began to have dreams of communion wafers crawling with insects, of pearls oozing mucous, of the pastor blowing up the church just as I was about to serve communion for the first time" (Disch & Avery, 2001, p. 214). Finally, as suggested earlier, CPSA is a violation of the individual's understanding of God as a loving being who ensures that bad things will not happen to good people.

Like an earthquake, CPSA is a desecration that creates spiritual havoc. The individual's entire spiritual edifice is shaken to its foundations. Some people are able to conserve the sacred in their lives through nontraditional channels, such as psychotherapy, talking to family or friends, and 12-step programs (McLaughlin, 1994). But many, if not most, enter a period of spiritual struggle, one that represents a fork in the road leading either to spiritual transformation or spiritual disengagement.

TRANSFORMATION

Virtually no one goes through life unscathed by major life stressors. Oftentimes, traumatic events trigger a process of struggle in which the individual wrestles with spiritual matters. Spiritual struggles can take three forms: struggles with the divine (e.g., feelings of anger, abandonment, or fear in relation to God), interpersonal struggles (e.g., religious tension and conflict with family, church members and leaders, denomination), and intrapsychic struggles (e.g., religious doubts, questions about dogma, conflicts between thoughts, feelings, and behaviors; Pargament, Murray-Swank, Magyar, & Ano, 2005). Survivors of CPSA may find themselves struggling with all three—the divine, the religious community, and internal conflicts and confusion.

What implications do spiritual struggles hold for health and well-being? On the one hand, we might assume that these signs of spiritual distress bode poorly for the long-term functioning of the individual. On the other hand, it could be argued that struggles are a prerequisite for growth. After all, the world's greatest religious figures, from Moses and Buddha to Mohammed and Jesus, experienced their own periods of spiritual struggle yet emerged steeled and strengthened from their ordeals. Empirical studies offer support for both points of view. Spiritual struggles have been tied both to poorer physical and mental health and to growth (see Pargament, Murray-Swank, et al., 2005, for a review).

Whether struggles lead to growth or to decline may depend, in part, on the individual's ability to transform his or her understanding of and approach to the sacred. Religious traditions offer their adherents a variety of methods to encourage fundamental transformation in their relationship with the sacred. These include rites of passage that facilitate a change in the sacred status of the individual, changes in the pathways people take to the sacred, and conversions to a different understanding of God or a different kind of sacred striving (Pargament, 1997). Survivors of sexual abuse, however, are more likely than victims of other traumas to look beyond traditional religious offerings in their search for spiritual transformation (see Flynn, 2008). For example, Fater and Mullaney (2000) interviewed seven survivors of CPSA and found that most had shifted the central spiritual focus of their lives from institutional religious involvement to the role of caring for others. The pathway to the sacred for many survivors takes many people outside of traditional religious systems. As one survivor of incest said, "Spirituality is more important to me now than religion" (Kane, Cheston, & Greer, 1993, p. 235).

Not all spiritual transformations are positive. People can shift from loving, protective representations of God to images of a punishing God who is disappointed and condemning, an abandoning God who leaves people in their time of need, or a malicious God who chooses to play with life in capricious ways. For example, Mart (2004) described one of his interviewees, a survivor of sexual abuse by a priest who "wept as he told me that he worries constantly about his sins, fears eternal damnation, and needs desperately to speak to a priest. However, he is so frightened by priests that he cannot confess or take communion" (p. 470). Many people experience negative spiritual transformation as the loss of what they held sacred: the loss of their sense of themselves as spiritual beings, the loss of their ability to celebrate sexuality, the loss of their faith in the trustworthiness of others, or the loss of their capacity to feel love and compassion. One survivor described the loss of his identity and religious vocation: "I never became a priest . . . I would have left high school, entered the seminary, finished college, and become a priest . . . I regret it because my whole life seems to have been a secret. Stay in control, that way no one can figure it out" (Disch & Avery, 2001, p. 214).

Some attempt to fill their spiritual vacuum with destructive objects of devotion (e.g., alcohol, drugs, promiscuity, or violence). For others, negative spiritual transformations lead eventually to spiritual disengagement. Childhood sexual abuse from a variety of sources has been associated with less religious practice among adults (e.g., Finkelhor, Hotaling, Lewis, & Smith, 1989). In fact, many survivors of CPSA leave the church entirely and relinquish their religious identities. Mart (2004) studied

25 male victims of CPSA and found that only one still identified as Catholic and attended services. However, it is important to stress that spiritual disengagement is not necessarily permanent. Spirituality has proven itself to be quite resilient to even the most traumatic of life events, such as the Holocaust (Brenner, 1980). Those who disengage then may eventually rediscover the sacred, but the process of recovery from CPSA and rediscovery of the sacred may be measured better in years and decades than days and months.

Once spirituality has been transformed or rediscovered, the individual engages anew in the process of conservation, sustaining and enhancing the sacred as it is now understood. In this sense, the search for the sacred—discovery, conservation, transformation—evolves continuously over the individual's lifespan. In this section, we have described the process of spirituality and the impact of CPSA on the spirituality of the survivor. It should be abundantly clear that survivors face difficult challenges in their spiritual journeys. For many survivors, spirituality is a part of the problem they are experiencing, yet spirituality can also serve as a valuable resource to many survivors. In the following section, we consider the practical implications of spirituality for treatment. More specifically, we examine how to address spirituality when it is a problem for the client and when it represents a potential solution to the client's problem.

CLINICAL IMPLICATIONS

Traditionally, mental health professionals have tended to overlook the spiritual dimension of human problems or "psychologize" this aspect of life. Neither approach is likely to be effective, especially in the context of CPSA. The problem of CPSA raises powerful spiritual issues that cry out for attention in any effective approach to treatment. Reducing struggles with God, church, or matters of faith to epiphenomena—expressions of something presumably more basic, such as unresolved conflicts with parents and authority figures—is also unlikely to help the client who experiences spiritual struggles as significant realities in and of themselves.

If the spiritual dimension should not be ignored or "explained away," how is it best addressed in the process of psychotherapy? A complete answer to this question would require a book and, in fact, a number of valuable texts have been written on religion, spirituality, and psychotherapy (e.g., Griffith & Griffith, 2002; Pargament, 2007; Propst, 1988; Richards & Bergin, 2005; Shafranske, 1996). In this section, we will briefly review three practical implications of a spiritually integrated approach to treating survivors of CPSA: creating a spiritual dialogue, accessing spiritual resources, and addressing spiritual problems. Following this review, we will examine one promising manualized spiritually integrated treatment program designed to work specifically with adults who experienced sexual abuse as children.

CREATING A SPIRITUAL DIALOGUE

Studies suggest that many clients, including those facing the most serious of problems, would be more than happy to talk about spiritual matters if clinicians were open to the topic (Lindgren & Coursey, 1995). It is not difficult to convey an interest in this dimension of life to clients. In the initial interview, the clinician can note, "We've talked about how the sexual abuse affected you physically, emotionally, and socially. I wonder how it might have affected you spiritually?" Embedded in this question is an invitation to the client to enter into a conversation about this potentially important but often neglected topic. Some clients may welcome the invitation and respond immediately with significant thoughts and feelings. Others may be more hesitant or unsure how to respond, perhaps because they are reluctant to share such personal information until they have formed a more trusting relationship with the therapist or perhaps because they are unaware of the role of spirituality in their lives. Thus, the clinician should remain alert to signs of spirituality even among clients who initially express disinterest in spiritual conversation. For example, ostensibly nonspiritual clients may draw on quasispiritual language to describe their experience of CPSA (e.g., "I felt desecrated," "When will my suffering end?" "I feel an emptiness in my soul"). By responding to this language with spiritual questions of his or her own, the therapist can facilitate surprising and important new conversation.

Spiritual dialogue is fostered by an open, curious attitude on the part of the clinician. It is not the therapist's place to criticize or proselytize the client's spiritual or nonspiritual orientation. Conversation is encouraged most importantly by the clinician's evident interest in learning more about the client's spiritual perspective. "Tell me more" is perhaps the most helpful of all questions. Remember though that spirituality, for many clients who have encountered CPSA, is an emotional landmine, a subject capable of eliciting the full range of explosive affects, from shame and despair to grief and anger. Listen, for example, to the rage one victim of incest voices to God:

How could you in all your greatness have abandoned me, a little girl, to the merciless hands of my father? How could you let this happen to me, I demand to know why this happened? Why didn't you protect me? I have been faithful, and for what, to be raped and abused by my own father? I hate and despise you. I regret the first time I ever laid eyes on you; your name is like salt on my tongue. I vomit it from my being. I wish death upon you. You are no more. You are dead. (Flaherty, 1992, p. 101)

These are powerful feelings, feelings that are often difficult for clients to admit and express, but they are not unusual to those who have experienced such a fundamental betrayal. The client, in this case, is following a time-honored tradition in religious circles—lamenting—a process of voicing anger toward God that may be a necessary step toward healing (Novotni, 2001). By accepting and normalizing the full range of spiritual emotions elicited by CPSA, the clinician can help lift the client's burden of spiritual shame and set the stage for positive spiritual transformation.

Through the spiritual conversation, the clinician also assesses where the client is in the search for the sacred. How does the client understand and experience the sacred? What pathways is the client taking to the sacred? Is the client in a process of discovery, conservation, struggle, transformation, or disengagement? And most important, how might spirituality be a part of the solution to the client's problems? How might spirituality be a problem in and of itself?

ACCESSING SPIRITUAL RESOURCES

Although CPSA can damage if not destroy many spiritual resources, other resources may remain intact and new ones may develop. Mental health professionals can assist their clients by helping them identify and draw on these remaining spiritual assets or new ones. Spiritual support represents one such potentially powerful resource. For example, in her book on spirituality for survivors of childhood sexual abuse, Flaherty (1992) described a number of visualization exercises she uses to help people gain spiritual support. In one exercise, she asks her female clients to sit in the place of Mary Magdalene weeping outside of the empty tomb of Jesus. The empty tomb, the woman is told, symbolizes all of the losses she has experienced. She is asked to imagine Jesus approaching her and asking, "Woman, why are you weeping?" (p. 56). The woman is encouraged to feel the presence and support of Jesus in her pain.

Biblical stories can also help people frame their suffering in a larger religious context (Schwartz & Kaplan, 1998). For instance, the story of slavery of the Hebrew people in Egypt and exodus to the Promised Land can place both the client's suffering and yearning for peace and freedom into a broader and, ultimately, more hopeful framework.

Rituals of purification can assist survivors of CPSA in replacing their feelings of contamination, shame, and guilt with a sense of spiritual cleansing and reconciliation. Testimony is an important part of the process of ritual purification, for it provides the client with an opportunity not only for catharsis but also to make meaning of, take control over, and experience dignity in one's own life narrative (Agger & Jensen, 1990). Therapists can help their clients "bear witness" to their pain by encouraging them to tell their stories. By responding to these stories with caring and acceptance rather than rejection and blame, clinicians may help many clients experience feelings of purification akin to religious confession. Among clients who can identify a trusted spiritual figure, the healing process could be promoted further by involvement in more formal confession and reconciliation rituals. For example, the organization Healing Voices, devoted to survivors of CPSA, offers a Service of Atonement where survivors, friends, and church leaders come together for healing and reconciliation.

Implicit in this latter point is the importance of helping survivors of CPSA distinguish between unsafe and safe clerical figures. Many survivors will not be able to make this kind of differentiation for many years, if ever. However, clinicians should not automatically assume that survivors of CPSA will have rejected religion in its entirety. With encouragement, many may be able to identify authentically committed religious figures who represent invaluable and perhaps unique sources of support. Consider, for example, the words of one survivor:

> Fortunately, I was blessed to trust a priest with my story, who instinctively knew that I needed even more than a psychiatrist could offer. This priest, Father A, has been able to pick up where my psychiatrist readily admits he could not go. There are some wounds that only God and Christ working through his people and his church can heal. Not only has Father A spoken to me tirelessly of God's love, but he alone has offered me healing through the sacraments. Last spring there were times when I believed I could not go on . . . I actually thought that driving my car into a brick wall would be

better than living this daily hell. Father A used his priesthood to offer me healing. His humility, his holiness, his sincerity, and his honest desire to help allowed me to accept what I probably would not have accepted from anyone else. (Smith, 2004, p. 9)

In short, although CPSA often leads to spiritual damage among survivors, other spiritual resources that continue to support and sustain the individual, or help the individual grow, may remain untouched. These resources will vary from person to person. The mention of God to one client may elicit deep feelings of bitterness and anger, while another may be deeply comforted by his or her religious faith. A ritual that triggers traumatic memories for one client may continue to hold a great deal of meaning for another. By helping clients identify and draw on their distinctive spiritual resources, mental health professionals can facilitate the process of healing.

ADDRESSING SPIRITUAL PROBLEMS

CPSA can strip old systems of spiritual belief and practice of their ability to generate spiritual meaning, comfort, or guidance for many survivors. When this occurs, spirituality becomes more a source of stress and strain than a source of solutions to problems. The yearning for the sacred may remain, but the client is unlikely to grow spiritually until these spiritual problems are addressed and a fundamental change takes place. Spiritually sensitive therapists can assist their clients in this process of spiritual transformation.

Many survivors of CPSA struggle with their representation of the sacred. Patriarchal images of God, so prevalent in the United States, may no longer be viable for those who have been abused by male clergy. Clinicians can help survivors seeking another way to envision a higher power. In this process of spiritual re-creation, the survivor may shift from the image of a distant God to a sacred power that lies within oneself, from a disinterested uncaring God to a compassionate deity, or from an all-powerful Father to a nurturant Mother. Flaherty (1992) suggested a number of images of an immanent God for survivors of sexual abuse:

God is part of us, suffers with us, joins in our weeping, becomes one with us as we suffer. God shares our brokenness. God does not watch us weep. God weeps with us. . . . The immanent God is not distant but is involved with our rhythms, our emotions, our dying and rising. . . . When we experience the immanent God, we begin to view God's relationship to our abuse in a new way. God did not stand by and do nothing as we experienced sexual abuse; rather God was one with us in this tragedy. As we were abused, so also was God broken and wounded. As we heal, God heals with us; as we become enraged as a result of our violation, so does God experience anger. (p. 109)

Similarly, Meehan (1991) provides people with a variety of ways to imagine God as a strong, empowering, feminine figure:

Imagine God as a Mother Eagle carrying you on her wing . . . empowering you with her strength . . . giving you the courage you need to be a risk-taker . . . challenging you to change unjust situations and structures . . . liberating you from every kind of oppression . . . filling you with love. (p. 21)

Clients may also need help in replacing old rituals, those that have become problematic by virtue of their association with a perpetrator of sexual abuse, with new and more vital rituals. Fortunately, there is no shortage of spiritual practices that can be adapted to the particular needs of clients. For example, though meditation may bring to mind the image of people sitting motionless in a lotus position for extended periods of time, this is only one of many forms of meditation (Wachholtz & Pargament, 2004). Meditation can also focus on the repetition of a meaningful meditative phrase (i.e., sacred meditation), reflection on a particular passage from a sacred text (i.e., devotional meditation), meditative singing and dancing, or walking through the sacred space of a labyrinth. Though these spiritual practices are quite varied, each is designed to help the client go beyond ordinary experience and the stresses of day-to-day life to deeper levels of the mind. Therapists can also help survivors of CPSA create their own distinctive rituals and spiritual narratives. As with meditation, these rituals can take a number of forms, but as a group, effective rituals have several common elements: they allow for the telling of a story of crisis, loss, and transition; they draw on nonverbal symbols as a way of expressing what words fail to express; they are tailored to the particulars of an individual's experience; and they tend to be simple rather than complicated (Anderson & Foley, 1998).

For example, in the spiritually integrated intervention we will review later, survivors of sexual abuse participate in a ritual titled the "Basket of

Shame" (Murray-Swank, 2003). In this ritual, survivors write down the "lies of shame" that they believe such as "I am worthless," "I caused the abuse to happen," "I am damaged," or "I am bad at the core of me." If they feel comfortable, clients are encouraged to speak these and other messages of shame out loud. Next, they rip up the pieces of paper, and place them in a Basket of Shame, which is filled with dirt, sticks, and stones representing the shame and areas of dryness in their lives that long for love and new life. After listening to a reflection and prayer on letting go of "the sticks and rocks we carry deep in our souls," a rose is placed in the Basket of Shame. A reflective prayer is then read about the rose of beauty, fullness, and spiritual worth that each individual carries within. Clients bring the roses home with them as a reminder of the true nature of their souls.

Finally, some survivors of abuse seek help in letting go of their intense feelings of anger, rage, and resentment toward their perpetrator, the larger religious institution, and the world more generally. Though these negative emotions are natural responses to the experience of sexual violation, they are not emotions that survivors have chosen for themselves. In the experience of emotional pain, many survivors feel they continue to be controlled and victimized by their perpetrators. Moving from anger to peace then represents a spiritually meaningful, empowering, transformational goal for at least some survivors (Pargament & Rye, 1998). It is important to stress that the process of letting go of anger should not be confused with forgetting the offense, condoning, exonerating, or reconciling with the perpetrator. The survivor can choose to develop greater mastery of his or her own emotions without minimizing the severity of the trauma.

It is important to consider a related but controversial topic—forgiveness. Some evidence suggests that forgiveness might be helpful to survivors of sexual abuse. Freedman and Enright (1996) evaluated the impact of a forgiveness intervention for 12 female incest survivors. Participants were assigned to the forgiveness intervention or a wait-list control. In contrast to the control group, the women who received the forgiveness intervention reported significantly greater gains in forgiveness and hope, and significantly greater reductions in anxiety and depression. Moreover, these gains were maintained when the treatment group was reexamined one year later. Though the results of this study of incest survivors were promising, we believe clinicians must be very cautious in using the language of forgiveness with survivors of sexual abuse. The term may be inappropriate for many survivors who believe that the concept delegitimates their natural feelings of bitterness and betrayal. Furthermore, forgiveness interventions are often based on the development of greater empathy for and sensitivity to perpetrators, a task that may be simply Herculean for most survivors. Finally, the concept of forgiveness may elicit feelings of guilt among survivors who feel unable to practice what is often described as a cardinal virtue in our culture. For these reasons, rather than broach the topic of forgiveness, we believe it is generally more helpful to speak to survivors about the shift from anger to peace or "letting go of anger" for their personal well-being.

In this section, we have illustrated some of the diverse ways clinicians can help their clients draw on their spiritual resources and address their spiritual problems. Though spiritual resources and spiritual problems are likely to vary from person to person, there are a number of spiritual issues that are prevalent among survivors of CPSA. Manualized treatment approaches could be developed that focus on these common spiritual resources and problems. We turn our attention now to one such promising program developed by Nichole Murray-Swank.

SOLACE FOR THE SOUL: FACILITATING SPIRITUAL TRANSFORMATION

Solace for the Soul: A Journey Towards Wholeness (Murray-Swank, 2003) is a spiritually integrated intervention that helps survivors of sexual abuse both conserve and transform the experience of the sacred in their lives. This intervention directly opens the door to an ongoing spiritual dialogue with survivors of sexual abuse, with the goals of accessing spiritual resources, and, in particular, addressing spiritual problems.

As mentioned earlier, CPSA may create a fertile environment for the process of spiritual growth and transformation. As survivors are stripped of old systems that no longer can be conserved in light of their experiences of CPSA, new grounds for transformation are cultivated. However, as discussed, this is unlikely to occur until spiritual problems and spiritual struggles are addressed. Therefore, one of the primary aims in the development of *Solace for the Soul* is to address the spiritual struggles that can result from experiences of sexual abuse and to enhance the process of spiritual transformation.

Broadly, *Solace for the Soul: A Journey Towards Wholeness* is an eight-session manualized intervention for individual clients that focuses on seven themes: images of God, spiritual journeys, abandonment and anger at God, spiritual connection, shame, the body, and sexuality (see

Murray-Swank, 2003; Murray-Swank & Pargament, 2005b). A 10-session group format is also available for the spiritually integrated intervention (Murray-Swank, 2002). *Solace for the Soul* is a nondenominational intervention that is rooted in a theistic, spiritual worldview similar to the one proposed by Richards and Bergin (2005). In general, this theistic perspective is consonant with the five major monotheistic world religions (Judaism, Christianity, Islam, Zoroastrianism, and Sikhism; Richards & Bergin, 2005). A trained therapist meets individually with each client for 1.5 hours each session. Overall, the spiritually integrated intervention includes opening and closing prayers, focused breathing, spiritual imagery, poems and reflection, two-way journaling to God, spiritual rituals, and discussion throughout the eight sessions.

More specifically, in Session 1, clients gain information about the program, discuss goals, and reflect on self-identified areas of strength and wholeness. For example, clients read the spiritual poem "The Weaver" (Foote, 1994) and reflect on the following quotes: "Out of the torn places, I reclaim wholeness. Out of the broken places, I reclaim strength." They write their responses to and discuss the following questions: "In what areas of my life do I desire wholeness? In what areas am I called to regain strength?" Session 2 focuses on clients' spiritual journeys and images of God. After clients "map" their spiritual journeys to date, they draw and describe current images of God. As discussed, masculine images of God may present challenges to those who have been abused by male clergy members and/or by males in general. Therefore, clients begin to reflect on and explore varied images of God, including immanent and feminine images of God. For example, clients participate in spiritual visualization exercises in which they imagine God's love as a waterfall within, God as a spirit of freedom, and God as a Mother eagle. Clients continue this work at home in between sessions.

In Session 3, clients begin the process of addressing their spiritual struggles surrounding their experiences of sexual abuse. First, feelings such as abandonment and anger at God are normalized, and clients read accounts of other survivors' spiritual struggles (e.g., Flaherty, 1992). Clients express their feelings of abandonment, anger, or spiritual disconnection and engage in a process of two-way journaling to God. In this exercise, clients write a letter to God and then "listen" for a reply and write the words or images they "hear." After beginning to express and work through their spiritual struggles, Session 4 focuses on enhancing a sense of spiritual connection with the sacred and with others (the "Vertical" and the "Horizontal"). Clients explore varied ways to connect to the presence of God in their lives and to enhance their spiritual connection with others. For example, a spiritual imagery exercise of divine light followed by a loving kindness meditation connects clients to the spiritual presence in their lives and to other survivors of sexual abuse.

Session 5 raises the issue of shame, as clients explore distorted cognitions about the self and use spiritual affirmations and rituals to reduce shame-based views. For example, clients write out the "lies of shame" such as "I am worthless/damaged/inadequate" and then write and focus on the voice of God's love including "I am sacred/lovable/not at fault." The spiritual ritual of the shame basket described previously is used to close this session. Expanding on the difficult work completed in this session, clients next focus on deeply held thoughts and feelings about the way sexual abuse impacted their bodies and sexuality in Sessions 6 and 7. Spiritual affirmations, cognitive restructuring, and journal reflections are used to reduce sexual dysfunction and body disparagement (e.g., body loathing). For example, clients consider the ways that sexual abuse shaped their thoughts about sex (e.g., "sex is shameful; sex is frightening") and consider alternate spiritual affirmations about sex (e.g., "sex is respectful; sex is sacred"). A primary goal of these sessions is to separate the abuse experiences from positive experiences of the body and sexuality, aiding in the transformation process.

Finally, Session 8 focuses on future directions and solidifying progress made in the spiritually integrated intervention. A spiritual ritual is used to highlight the strengths, courage, and vibrancy of each survivor of sexual abuse. This includes a bouquet of flowers used to represent each person the client knows who has experienced sexual abuse. The flowers are placed in a vase by both the client and the therapist, and a poem and reflection are read to close the intervention, focused on the growth, healing, and spiritual transformation of each survivor.

A pilot research study on the effectiveness of *Solace for the Soul: A Journey Towards Wholeness* yielded promising results (Murray-Swank & Pargament, 2005a, 2005b). Upon entering the program for this study, some survivors were searching for a way to conserve their spiritualities in the midst of coping with the long-term effects of childhood incest, and for some, additional clergy abuse. In the words of one survivor of CPSA: "The abuse by my pastor destroyed my faith. I needed to leave that denomination . . . yet my belief in God never wavered." This client conserved her image of God and personal relationship with God, yet transformed her religious belief system, practices, and denomination. In the words of another survivor: "God was always there for me. The only one . . . the one I turned to all those years. I always relied on God." As a survivor of severe childhood satanic ritual abuse, this client entered the program searching to strengthen her spiritual life, stating, "I want to strengthen my relationship with God . . . not just when times are bad, but all the time." In these examples, the survivors of sexual abuse sought to build on and maintain their relationship with the sacred in their lives.

Other participants began the program in the midst of spiritual upheaval and struggle. No longer able to conserve their spirituality or old systems of beliefs, they were seeking transformation. For example, one client said, "I hope to gain a better understanding of abuse and God. Why He abandoned me and why I can't feel Him beside me now . . . I want a relationship with God back." This process of spiritual transformation can be difficult and painful, yet ultimately rewarding. In the previous example, this female survivor of sexual abuse transformed her beliefs about God's responsibility in the abuse, changing from anger at God to spiritual connection. At the end of the spiritually integrated intervention she declared, "I know now that God is not the person to be angry at. I am angry at the person *who's fault it is* . . . my dad. I am on my way." Another client experienced a connection with God for the first time, and changed her image of God from a distant, impersonal, and absent God to a God whom she described as supportive, gentle, guiding, and giving (see Murray-Swank & Pargament, 2005a for more details). In general, substantial spiritual transformations occurred for those in the midst of spiritual struggles.

The empirical results of this study highlighted both the psychological and spiritual transformation that can be achieved through a spiritually integrated intervention for survivors of sexual abuse. For example, the participants demonstrated significant decreases in psychological distress and psychopathology (e.g., depression, anxiety) in the long term (i.e., 1 to 2 month follow-up). In addition, the majority experienced a reduction in their trauma symptoms across the course of the intervention and at a 1 to 2 month follow-up. Finally, those clients who entered the program in the midst of spiritual struggles demonstrated increases in their use of positive religious coping, spiritual well-being, and positive images of God across time and at the follow-up period (see Murray-Swank & Pargament, 2005b).

In summary, *Solace for the Soul: A Journey Towards Wholeness* (Murray-Swank, 2003) encourages a spiritual dialogue that is frequently neglected in trauma treatment. In addition, it provides an avenue for survivors of CPSA, and other survivors of sexual abuse, to address the spiritual problems and struggles that frequently lead to spiritual disengagement and poor psychological health. Finally, it opens the door to spiritual transformation, re-creation, and growth. In the words of one survivor, "Like a sunflower, I have opened and reached out towards the sun."

CONCLUSION

Researchers and practitioners are only beginning to learn about the spiritual dimension of CPSA. What we do know, however, is that CPSA is not simply a psychological, social, or physical event; it is a spiritual trauma. In their assessment of the damage that results from CPSA, clinicians should be sure to attend to the spiritual dimension. Progress in psychotherapy may rest on the clinician's willingness to address the spiritual problems created by sexual abuse. Yet spirituality can be a source of solutions as well as a source of problems. Therapeutic progress can also be facilitated by the clinician's willingness to help clients identify and draw on their spiritual resources. Perhaps the greatest challenge for mental health professionals is to become better acquainted with the multifaceted nature of spiritual life, both the bitter and the sweet. Formal course training, continuing education, and advanced clinical supervision in the domain of spirituality are all important prerequisites to practice in this area. Equally important is the clinician's openness to learning about the place of spirituality in the lives of clients and in the life of the therapist himself or herself. With a deeper knowledge of spirituality, therapists will be better equipped to integrate this dimension of life more fully into the process of healing.

REFERENCES

Agger, I., & Jensen, S. B. (1990). Testimony as ritual and evidence as psychotherapy for political refugees. *Journal of Traumatic Stress, 3,* 115–130.

Anderson, H., & Foley, E. (1998). *Mighty stories, dangerous rituals: Weaving together the human and the divine.* San Francisco: Jossey-Bass.

Ano, G. A., & Vasconcelles, E. B. (2005). Religious coping and psychological adjustment to stress: A meta-analysis. *Journal of Clinical Psychology, 61,* 461–480.

Anonymous. (1990). An adult survivor of child abuse speaks up. In S. J. Rosetti (Ed.), *Slayer of the soul: Child sexual abuse and the Catholic Church* (pp. 113–122). Mystic, CT: Twenty-Third Publications.

Bouchard, R. J., Jr., Lykken, D. T., McGue, M., Segal, N. L., & Tellegen, A. (1990). Sources of human psychological differences: The Minnesota study of twins reared apart. *Science, 250,* 223–250.

Brenner, R. (1980). *The faith and doubt of Holocaust survivors.* New York: Free Press.

Brother Lawrence. (1975). *Practice of the presence of God.* Nashville: Abingdon.

Browne, A., & Finkelhor, D. (1986). Impact of child sexual abuse: A review of the research. *Psychological Bulletin, 99*, 66–77.

Chibnall, J. T., Wolf, A., & Duckro, P. N. (1998). A national survey of the sexual trauma experiences of Catholic nuns. *Review of Religious Research, 40*, 142–167.

Coles, R. (1990). *The spiritual life of children*. Boston: Houghton Mifflin.

Disch, E., & Avery, N. (2001). Sex in the consulting room, the examining room, and the sacristy: Survivors of sexual abuse by professionals. *American Journal of Orthopsychiatry, 71*, 204–217.

Durkheim, E. (1915). *The elementary forms of the religious life*. New York: Free Press.

Emmons, R. A. (1999). *The psychology of ultimate concerns: Motivation and spirituality in personality*. New York: Guilford.

Exline, J. J., Yali, A. M., & Lobel, M. (1999). When God disappoints: Difficulty forgiving God and its role in negative emotion. *Journal of Health Psychology, 4*, 365–379.

Fater, K., & Mullaney, J. A. (2000). The lived experience of adult male survivors who allege childhood sexual abuse by clergy. *Issues in Mental Health Nursing, 21*, 281–295.

Finkelhor, D., Hotaling, G. T., Lewis, I. A., & Smith, C. (1989). Sexual abuse and its relationship to later sexual satisfaction, marital status, religion, and attitudes. *Journal of Interpersonal Violence, 4*, 379–399.

Fitchett, G., Rybarczyk, B. D., DeMarco, G. A., & Nicholas, J. J. (1999). The role of religion in rehabilitation outcomes: A longitudinal study. *Rehabilitation Psychology, 44*, 1–22.

Flaherty, S. M. (1992). *Woman, why do you weep? Spirituality for survivors of childhood sexual abuse*. New York: Paulist Press.

Flynn, K. A. (2008). In their own voice: Women who were sexually abused by members of the clergy. *Journal of Child Sexual Abuse, 17*(3–4), 216–237.

Foote, C. (1994). *Survivor prayers: Talking with God about childhood sexual abuse*. Louisville, KY: Westminster/John Knox Press.

Freedman, S. R., & Enright, R. D. (1996). Forgiveness as an intervention goal with incest survivors. *Journal of Consulting and Clinical Psychology, 64*, 983–992.

Griffith, J. L., & Griffith, M. E. (2002). *Encountering the sacred in psychotherapy: How to talk with people about their spiritual lives*. New York: Guilford Press.

Johnson, P. E. (1959). *Psychology of religion*. Nashville, TN: Abingdon Press.

Kane, D., Cheston, S. E., & Greer, J. (1993). Perceptions of God by survivors of childhood sexual abuse: An exploratory study in an underresearched area. *Journal of Psychology and Theology, 21*, 228–237.

Kaufman, G. D. (1981). *The theological imagination: Constructing the concept of God*. Philadelphia: Westminster.

Koenig, H. G., McCullough, M. E., & Larson, D. B. (2001). *Handbook of religion and health*. New York: Oxford University Press.

Lindgren, K. N., & Coursey, R. D. (1995). Spirituality and serious mental illness: A two-part study. *Psychosocial Rehabilitation Journal, 18*, 93–111.

Mahoney, A., Pargament, K. I., Ano, G., Lynn, Q., Magyar, G. M., McCarthy, S., et al. (2002, August). *The devil made them do it? Demonization and the 9/11 attacks*. Paper presented at the Annual Meeting of the American Psychological Association, Chicago, IL.

Mart, E. G. (2004). Victims of abuse by priests: Some preliminary observations. *Pastoral Psychology, 52*, 465–472.

Matchan, L. (1992, June 8). Ex-priest's accusers tell of the damage. *Boston Globe*, pp. 1, 8.

McLaughlin, B. R. (1994). Devastated spirituality: The impact of clergy sexual abuse on the survivor's relationship with God and the church. *Sexual Addiction and Compulsivity, 1*, 145–158.

Meehan, B. M. (1991). *Exploring the feminine face of God: A prayerful journey.* New York: Sheed and Ward.

Murray-Swank, N. A. (2002). *Solace for the soul: A group psycho-spiritual intervention for female survivors of sexual abuse.* Unpublished treatment manual, Bowling Green, OH.

Murray-Swank, N. A. (2003). *Solace for the soul: A journey towards wholeness. Treatment manual for female survivors of sexual abuse.* Baltimore, MD: Loyola College.

Murray-Swank, N. A., & Pargament, K. I. (2005a). God, where are you? Evaluating a spiritually-integrated intervention for sexual abuse. *Mental Health, Religion, and Culture, 8*, 191–204.

Murray-Swank, N. A., & Pargament, K. I. (2005b). *Solace for the soul: Evaluating spiritually-integrated psychotherapy for survivors of sexual abuse.* Manuscript submitted for publication.

Novotni, M. (2001). *Angry with God.* Colorado Springs, CO: New Press.

Pargament, K. I. (1997). *The psychology of religion and coping: Theory, research, practice.* New York: Guilford Press.

Pargament, K. I. (1999). The psychology of religion and spirituality? Yes and no. *The International Journal for the Psychology of Religion, 9*, 3–16.

Pargament, K. I. (2007). *Spiritually integrated psychotherapy: Understanding and addressing the sacred.* New York: Guilford Press.

Pargament, K. I., Koenig, H. G., Tarakeshwar, N., & Hahn, J. (2001). Religious struggle as a predictor of mortality among medically ill elderly patients: A two-year longitudinal study. *Archives of Internal Medicine, 161*, 1881–1885.

Pargament, K. I., Magyar, G. M., Benore, E., & Mahoney, A. (2005). Sacrilege: A study of sacred loss and desecration and their implications for health and well-being in a community sample. *Journal for the Scientific Study of Religion, 44*, 59–78.

Pargament, K. I., & Mahoney, A. (2002). Spirituality: Discovering and conserving the sacred. In C. R. Snyder & S. J. Lopez (Eds.), *Handbook of positive psychology* (pp. 646–659). Oxford: Oxford University Press.

Pargament, K. I., & Mahoney, A. (2005). Sacred matters: Sanctification as a vital topic for the psychology of religion. *The International Journal for the Psychology of Religion, 15*, 179–199.

Pargament, K. I., Murray-Swank, N., Magyar, G., & Ano, G. (2005) Spiritual struggle: A phenomenon of interest to psychology and religion. In W. R. Miller & H. Delaney (Eds.), *Judeo-Christian perspectives on psychology: Human nature, motivation, and change* (pp. 245–268). Washington DC: APA Press.

Pargament, K. I., & Rye, M. (1998). Forgiving as a method of religious coping. In E. Worthington & M. McCullough (Eds.), *Dimensions of forgiveness: Psychological research and theological perspectives* (pp. 59–78). Philadelphia: Templeton Press.

Propst, R. L. (1988). *Psychotherapy in a religious framework.* New York: Human Sciences Press.

Richards, P. S., & Bergin, A. E. (2005). *A spiritual strategy for counseling and psycho-therapy*. Washington DC: American Psychological Association.

Rizzuto, A. M. (1979). *The birth of the living God: A psychoanalytic study*. Chicago: University of Chicago Press.

Rosetti, S. J. (1995). The impact of child sexual abuse on attitudes toward God and the Catholic church. *Child Abuse and Neglect, 19*, 1469–1481.

Schwartz, M. B., & Kaplan, K. J. (1998). Self-esteem: Strengths, gifts, and healing. *Journal of Psychology and Judaism, 22*, 161–174.

Shafranske, E. P. (Ed.). (1996). *Religion and the clinical practice of psychology*. Washington DC: American Psychological Association.

Smith, M. (2004). A survivor's story. *Human Development, 1*, 5–10.

Valentine, L., & Feinauer, L. L. (1993). Resilience factors associated with female survivors of childhood sexual abuse. *The American Journal of Family Therapy, 21*, 216–224.

Wachholtz, A., & Pargament, K. I. (2004). Spiritual meditation as a resource for troubled parishioners. In D. Herl & M. L. Berman (Eds.), *Building bridges over troubled waters: Enhancing pastoral care and guidance* (pp. 276–291). Lima, OH: Wyndham Hall Press.

Index

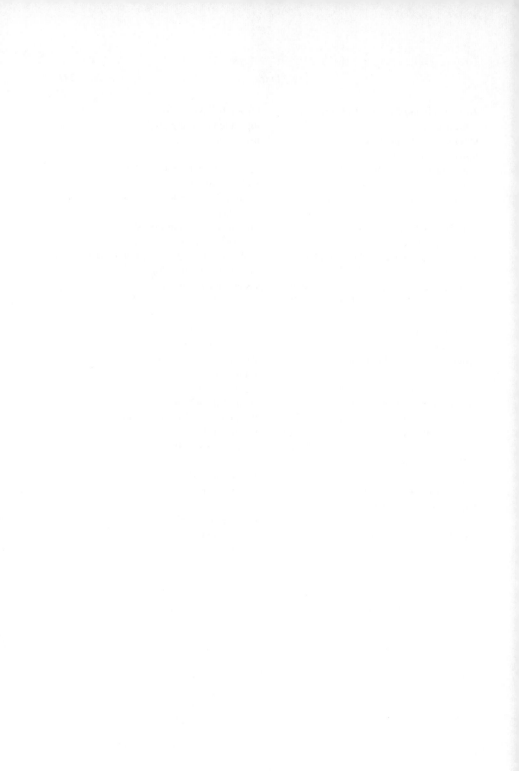